IT'S NEVER TOO LATE

Dr. Ed Wolfgram's Book of Fitness

TO my Susan
Good Health to you
Ed Wolfgram
Ironman Champion
1st Place 2003
age 70-74 group.

twice 2nd
twice 4th.

IT'S NEVER TOO LATE

Dr. Ed Wolfgram's Book of Fitness

By Ed and Dorothea Wolfgram with
research assistance from
Tim Meyer, Ph.D. candidate

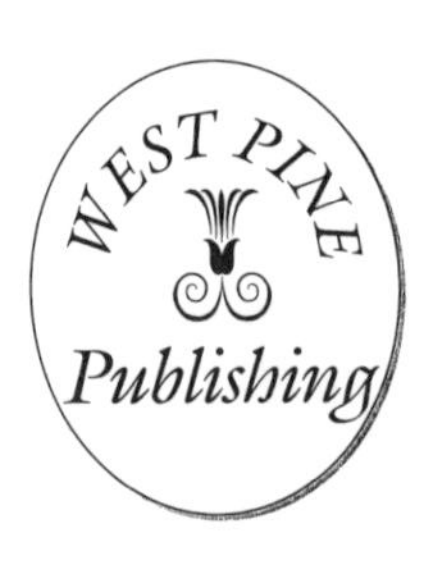

www.fitness-never2late.com

Published by West Pine Press
4500 West Pine Boulevard
St. Louis, Missouri 63108

Cover photo by Andy Mannis, Madison, Wisconsin
Back cover photo by Dryfus & Associates, photographers
Book design by Shirin Ardakani

ISBN 0-9701420-1-3

To our parents and children and to the wonderful athletes who are our support community.

Contents

Chapter 1

Why?

Ed Wolfgram always opens his talks on fitness by saying,

"Remember, it is never too late. When I was 48, I couldn't run to the end of the block. I looked around at my contemporaries and became frightened. They were suffering heart attacks and strokes, developing diabetes. Some were dying; some had died.

"My wife and I had married at 33. We had three children under 12; I couldn't afford to die or be disabled. And I certainly didn't want to.

"So I ran half a block the first day and a block the next. Fifteen months later and 25 pounds lighter, I ran a marathon. But I didn't train smart and I didn't run smart. I ran on sheer guts and fear. Don't do that.

"Right now, start to use your body more; but use it to give you the greatest benefits. One of an Ironman's secrets is that he or she swims, bikes, runs, and does weight training.

"That balance makes it possible for human beings to do an Ironman in Hawaii: To swim 2.4 miles in the ocean, bike 112 in the heat on a black road in a black lava field, and run 26.2 miles over the same road. But often, by the run, we are returning to the starting point in complete darkness.

"Until 2003, the World Championship Ironman date was set by the October full moon. Only elite competitors finish in daylight. The gun sounds at 7 a.m. The sun sets 12 hours later. Of the 1500 participants, fewer than half have crossed the finish line by that time.

"Nonindustrial Hawaii is very dark; we need the moonlight. Yet out there at the end of a long, long day, orientation is tough. You focus on the motion of a light wand someone has handed you. There is no traffic, the light reflectors that outline the road like a video game don't work. There is you—putting one foot down in front of the other—and the soft padding of other competitors. Some are just going out; you are glad you are not with them. You concentrate on not letting anyone pass you, on passing others.

"If you have run the race right, you are dead tired. Your only salvation is that others may be in worse shape. But you've been there before, you know you'll finish; time is the question. In the dark, in the weariness, you could pass your brother and not recognize him. You simply don't know, at that point, where your competitors are.

"It's too late to worry about that. You've trained your best; you've run a good race; trophying was the goal, but that's icing on the cake. You've done this for healthfulness. Push on to the end.

"For my age-group competitors that takes more than 14 hours. The pros do it in eight, start to finish. The last 7 a.m. starters stagger across the finish line just before midnight. Spectators are there in number to cheer them in. Every one of them is a winner.

"You can be too. Maybe you won't do the Ironman, but remember, even at 50 that's not an impossible goal. It takes will and way. I can teach you the way."

No one is too young or old to benefit from a resolve to take better care of the amazing, wonderful, miraculous body we have been endowed with by our creator. It is never too late to start.

AT 20

Our body is at a peak in our 20s. It is so perfectly made, so built for the long haul, so tolerant of our indulgences that almost nothing short of catastrophic trauma or abuse can damage it permanently.

We can live on hamburgers and pizza without heartburn. We can breathe our polluted air without panting. We can be weekend athletes and recover on Monday.

AT 30

By our 30s, that's no longer as true as we'd like to believe. We are losing muscle mass (as much as 10% a decade) and brain cells. Yet our creator designed us with such overcapacity, those losses aren't noticeable, yet.

Don't be fooled, however. The 30s can be dangerous. We are so busy raising a family, getting ahead at work, securing our future, we think we don't have time for exercise. Yet staying healthy is important to all of the above.

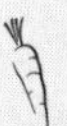

The current buzz is to replace the word *exercise* with the word *movement.* That may be good, but it's not for us (authors and readers). Even if you are 90, moving is good, exercise is better. In our civilized, sedentary world, it's a rare human who moves enough in ordinary, everyday life to stay fit.

AT 40

If the 30s *can be* dangerous, the 40s *are*.

We've picked up weight since high school. Now it's become too much. It has not only accumulated, it has settled around our middle. That's a very dangerous place. Our body put it there because we gave it excess food and it's storing that as fat in a secure place. It thinks it may need the fat to make energy in a time of famine. (In the past million years that's what it learned to do to survive. It will take humankind another million to teach our body not to hoard fat.)

To be failsafe, it put its emergency stores in a place that is hard to get to through movement. Even people who exercise vigorously can develop that spare tire. It's the first place we put on weight (women also tend to store fat in their thighs) and the last place we lose it.

What you need to do first is stop adding to your weight. Don't consume more calories than you use. Cut your caloric intake, increase your caloric output—move more to use more calories.

If we have not eaten right and not exercised—even if we abstained from smoking and excess alcohol—by the 40s we begin to fall victim to diseases of degeneration and lifestyle.

Fat has clogged our blood vessels, strained our heart, starved our brain of blood. Inactivity has allowed our muscles to lose strength and flexibility. Bone loss begins to invade areas of joint weakness from old sports injuries: all of us—men and women—complain of painful knees, elbows, shoulders.

AT 50

In our 50s all of these problems increase. Carrying around too much weight causes low back problems; arthritis invades our joints; stress disrupts our sleep and our digestion. Even

LISTEN UP!

Why do we tolerate being unhealthy or deteriorating with age?

We* determine what we weigh, how healthy our heart is (even with congenital heart disease), how strong and flexible our muscles are, how solid our bones are, how healthy our lungs are, how well our stomach, intestines, liver, kidneys, even sex organs function. We don't determine these by taking pills, we determine them by *lifestyle.

our sex drive suffers. No wonder we become depressed; we are falling apart. Barring disabling illness, our healthfulness is within our control. It depends largely on our lifestyle.

> Are we active or sedentary?

> Do we practice prevention, as prescribed by modern medicine?

> Do we eat healthfully and control our weight?

> Do we exercise routinely and do some strength training?

Staying healthy well into our 80s is very simple. There are two hard and fast rules:

> Stay active

> Eat right

In a 1996 federal government report, Donna Shalala, secretary of health and human services, says:

"This report is a passport to good health for all Americans. Its key finding is that people of all ages can improve the quality of their lives through a lifelong practice of moderate physical activity. You don't have to be training for the Boston Marathon to derive real health benefits from physical activity. A regular—preferably daily—regime of at least 30-45 minutes of brisk walking, bicycling, or even working around the house or yard will reduce your risks of developing coronary heart disease, hypertension, colon cancer, and diabetes. And if you are already doing that, you should consider picking up the pace: this report says that people who are already physically active will benefit even more by increasing the intensity or duration of their activity.

"This watershed report comes not a moment too soon. We have found that 60%—well over half—of Americans are not regularly active. Worse yet, 25% are not active at all. For young people—the future of our country—physical activity declines dramatically during adolescence. These are dangerous trends. We need to turn them around quickly, for the health of our citizens and our country....

"We Americans always find the will to change when change is needed...."

Many health and fitness books cite the gruesome and frightening statistics about the poor general health of the American people. We'll quote those statistics and cite those studies at various points. But, not here.

We prefer success stories and as Americans we have succeeded in the past 40 years. Paradoxically, we have also failed: we eat less fat, we are fatter; we do more invasive medical procedures, we haven't much extended life after illness onset; we exercise more, but not enough; we still don't eat right, but sometimes that's because we were misguided —and still are.

DON'T TRY, DO IT!

Remember four Ed Wolfgram guidelines:

> *More is always better.*
>
> If you can become an exercise fanatic, do. If you can't, do absolutely as much as you can. Just go easy at first. Every added effort brings more preventive health rewards.

> *Fit activity into your real life now. Don't wait for the perfect time or place.*
>
> In some ways, less can be good. You don't have to fall exhausted to your workout room floor to gain success.

Walk, ride a bike, cut the lawn, vacuum the living room, chase the kids or a golf ball, play tennis, skate, run, climb stairs. Start now, right where you are in life.

> *Find 30 ways in your everyday life to exercise. Put in as much time as you can eke out right now.*

Think about it; write the ways down. Every determined soul can use his/her body more. If you haven't two hours, patch together exercise in increments as short as 10 minutes.

To start with, get up earlier. I know of no Ironman whose day doesn't start before 6 a.m. with exercise. With family or even just a spouse, it's easier to find time at the beginning of the day, than in the middle or at the end. If you can't spare 30 minutes at lunch or before or after work for a run, a workout, a swim (because vigorous exercise also requires a shower and change of clothes) squeeze out small, less vigorous activity.

Walk or bike to work or to public transit. Walk to a restaurant or the park to brownbag. Park at the far end of any lot; walk the family to McDonald's. Climb stairs instead of taking an elevator or escalator. Walk any errand that doesn't require carrying lots of stuff to and from. Get off the bus a stop early, catch it a stop later on your route. Even, heaven forbid, give up the remote.

Do all of these little things, then block out some major time as often as you can. In total, this will increase your weekly activity immensely.

> *When you have downtime, fill it with exercise for your head, not your heart.*

Play bridge or poker; read; listen to music or words; argue politics, sports, movies; do a crossword puzzle; read to the kids or grandkids; play a game with them; surf the net; watch something live and/or challenging. Even when you are suffering from absolute feet-on-the-coffee-table fatigue, don't put up with mind pap. The latest Alzheimer's research proves that the brain—as well as the biceps—is an organ that benefits from exercise.

GET HEALTHY / STAY HEALTHY

The most commonly cited barrier to exercise is lack of time. That's a cop out.

It's also a gross misconception of priorities. The prize belongs to those who finish the race. A healthier you will be more alive mentally, as well as physically, will stay healthy when others begin to fail, will outlast the competition.

The most common reason for quitting physical activity—and this lesson may be the most important Ironman secret of all—is injury.

Three quick rules:

> Never use a sport that requires quick turns or jumps (and falls) as a primary activity (better golf than tennis, skating than basketball, volleyball or hockey). Good lord, don't quit sports you enjoy. Just don't be excessive. Those jerks and falls lead to injury.

> Always follow the Ironmen: cross-train. The traditional swim, bike, run uses and strengthens different sets of muscles, but you can make your own choices. Walk, swim, blade; row, bike, skate; play tennis, golf, swim; make up other combinations.

> Always do resistance training. In this, work on weak links, such as the neck, and strengthen muscles that oppose those you build in your exercise routine. Target opposing sets of muscles by specific isotonic or isometric training. Use abdominal sets to oppose back problems; stretches to oppose tightening; other isometrics to build wrist,

knee, elbow, shoulder overuse opposition. (You can design your own regime, but, in the beginning, it's better to get help from an expert in physiology. Insist that a trainer or a sport physiologist recommend regimes tailored to keep you—specifically you—injury free.)

NOW IS THE TIME

Be assured that retirement will not be golden or bring a renaissance of activity to those who haven't developed a commitment to health prior to those years.

Our favorite senior is a woman who never owned a car, always lived in the city and walked everywhere. Well into her 80s, she walked five miles a day doing routine rounds. When she relocated to Ohio, she joined the Appalachian Mountain Club to hike, as well as walk errands. At 97 she is giving up her home and entering a retirement village, but won't consider one that doesn't have an exercise room and regular physical activity program. At 75, we walked onto a playground where some 12-year-olds were jumping rope. She jumped into a set of double-Dutch.

Of course, her mental attitude matches her physical prowess. For her, life is still full of promise; she has little forbearance for a can't-do attitude.

Ed Wolfgram says, "As a physician of 40 years, I have never had a physically active person of any age walk into my psychiatric office with a depression.

"In contrast, as a forensic psychiatrist who often deals with legal cases arising from severe physical injury and lingering pain, I seldom have patients who are not depressed. They cannot move without pain. Without movement, their mental, as well as their physical, health deteriorates.

"Physical and mental health are always linked."

To be a promising workaholic at 30 whose energy is sapped by excessive weight, worry, and fatigue isn't likely to lead to the same "promising" designation at 40, to the executive suite at 50, or the seat at the head of the table at 60. For the fit, the competitive ranks will be thinned all along the career path by disabling illness and death.

Time spent keeping fit pays enormous economic—as well as social—rewards.

Chapter 2

Evolution and the Wondrous Us

The evolutionary history of the human body abhors sloth. It's a hard fact. We can't be sedentary and healthy. Exercise is vital.

Our body evolved for a life that demanded work from dawn to dusk. It evolved to deal with feast and famine—more famine than feast. Until the 20th century, being inactive was the option only of royalty. If common folk were to keep themselves clothed and fed, they had no significant relief from hard work. Today, few of us do hard physical labor routinely, but that is the mode of operation our every cell is programmed to expect.

As Ironmen (and women), we've reverted to our origins. Every person who completes the Ironman-distance race trains for hours—if not daily, at least four times a week. In doing so, we are using our bodies as they evolved to be used.

In a few million years, perhaps our body will adapt to be all brain and little brawn, but it cannot now. To be healthy we need to stress the body, to demand more of it than our normal daily lives require. We need to exercise.

In addition, to feed ourselves properly in *our* everyday world, we have to accommodate to our evolutionary mode of feast and famine. Should we gorge ourselves this week and starve ourselves the next? That's not recommended, but to eat right, we do need to take into account that history.

Because of it, our body learned to store excess calories in times of feast and to live off of them in times of famine. When we have excess calories all the time (as we do every day in America), our body puts those calories into storage. Its most efficient means of storage is *fat,* so it deposits fat stores all over the body.

Since we seldom experience famine, those stores are never tapped. The more we put into them, the more they accumulate. Our body has no shut-off valve. It never says, "Enough is enough, let's stop the storing." It always believes famine may be right around the corner. There are subtle ways to cut fat storage—which we'll recommend later—but no other natural methods decrease it.

Absolutely every diet is founded on three possible solutions or their combinations. All of them use stored fat to produce the energy for daily living.

- **Starve; Don't give the body the calories it needs to function normally;**
- **Exercise; use more calories than you are taking in;**
- **Trick the body into believing it is starving (by limiting intake of carbohydrates—the body's preferred source of energy) so it taps stored fat for energy.**

HARD WORK BUILDS HEALTHY HEARTS

One of the first long-term studies of coronary heart disease and exercise was done among 3686 longshoreman in San Francisco by Ralph Paffenbarger of Stanford University. He and his colleagues looked for the key to heart health among these men who hoisted, carried, and lowered heavy loads routinely during their work day.

Perhaps not unexpectedly, investigators found that a good many of their subjects smoked, drank, and, in leisure, sat around playing poker or watching television. Yet for all of these unhealthy habits, the incidence of heart attacks among them was as much as 49% lower than the age-adjusted national average.

In the same study, nonsmokers had a 30% lower incidence of heart disease than smokers. Scientists concluded that the hard physical labor of their subjects built a heart so strong that, on average, it withstood even the negative behaviors.

Clearly activity to the point of strain is essential to heart-health (and much other health). To be physically fit at almost any age, you need to challenge your body routinely.

Fitness has everything to do with the quality of your life now and forever. It bestows countless economic blessings. You will earn more over your working life and stay in line for advancement. It can lengthen your working life or give you a productive retirement.

HEALTH AND AGING

We can't claim that age is kind to the body. It isn't. It extracts an inevitable toll.

Hard as they train, Ironman competitors in every age group are slower than those five years younger. It is why in any group over 50, winners tend to be at the bottom of that five-year age group. It's why we wonder so at 30+-year-old Olympic contenders or professional athletes.

It is also why a competitor who unexpectedly dominates a group (in the youth-oriented Olympic competition or professional sports) is suspected of using performance-enhancing drugs, blood doping methods (doping increases the amount of oxygen the blood carries), or lying about his/her age.

It's why in the Hawaiian Ironman competition, anyone who dominates an age group to a remarkable degree may have his/her age or use of performance-enhancing drugs questioned. Athletes know that among the rest of them—despite their elite status—age is an egalitarian leveler.

Every recent study of exercise and aging (and in the past decade there have been hundreds) proves that you are never too old to reap the benefits of increased exercise. Studies that engaged 90-year-old nursing home patients in regular regimens of movement and resistance training (push against stress) show that, over the study period, subjects increased both muscle mass and strength.

Think of what that means in terms of overall health and longevity! One of the inevitable results of aging is a loss of lean muscle mass. (The scientific term for this is *sarcopenia.*)

Our body is composed of three types of muscle—cardiac (the heart), smooth muscle (the linings of many organs such as the stomach and the intestines) and skeletal. Skeletal muscle makes up a whopping 40% of our body. It provides for movement, postural support and—strangely—heat generation in times of cold stress (shivering). (Think about it, the chills of "chills and fever" are the body's way of shaking us up to heat us up.)

Skeletal muscles are attached to our bony skeleton by tendons. This delicate, vastly complicated, yet wonderfully enduring and forgiving system of leverage—skeletal muscle, tendon, cartilage, and bone—is in constant use, even as we sleep. Yet, unless we unbalance it or allow it to deteriorate by disuse, it works smoothly and efficiently for a century or more.

MUSCLE MASS AND STRENGTH

The muscle mass we lose in aging is almost all skeletal muscle. How much of it we lose depends on whether we use it or we don't. If we are active, we do. If we are sedentary, we don't. It's as simple as that.

Since muscles attach to bones (the points of attachment are the *origin*—where the muscle attaches to a relatively stable skeletal part, such as a joint—and the *insertion*—where the muscle attaches to a moving bone) keeping muscles active, keeps bones moving. That—and good nutrition—makes for healthy bones as well.

Think of what having more and stronger muscles means in terms of aging: It means that moving is easier and we do more of it. It means that bones are healthier and we are less likely to injure them, even in falls. It means that in movement we need more energy and our basal metabolic rate (how fast or slow our body uses energy) remains high. It means that since we need more energy, we can eat more and not get fat.

The opposite—losing lean muscle mass—has the same effect except that this one is a downward spiral. We lose muscle mass, we reduce our activity level, we decrease our basal metabolic rate, we decrease our energy requirement. We eat too much, exchange more muscle for fat, grow fat, move less, become tired more easily, can't do many of the things we once prized. We grow bored; if we don't die, we sometimes wish we would because life is so limited and miserable.

We once thought that degenerative diseases like heart disease, high blood pressure, strokes, diabetes, and senility were the inevitable consequences of aging. Our ancestors didn't have them simply because most of them didn't live that long. Yet, even though we believed this, all of us knew some octogenarians who lived active lives and had sound, healthy minds. If we bothered to wonder why, we discovered that most of them had worked hard and long in youth and mid-life.

Ed's mother, who lived *alone* well into her 90s and died at 100, was the eldest of five girls born into an Iowa farm family. Since he had no sons, her father made her his farm-hand. While her sisters cleaned the barn, tended the chickens, cooked and cleaned, she hitched up four horses, drove the team and plowed.

When she married and bore children, she continued to be her husband's farmhand, as well as his wife and the mother of their children. Every year she gardened, canned, and mothered her five children, a couple of hundred chickens and litters of piglets. Although she ran her household smoothly, she always preferred outside work. She worked hard from dawn to dusk. When they retired from farming and moved into town, she and her husband continued to work full time at other occupations.

Her husband died of an infection at 60, but she continued to raise other people's children to 77. Then she retired, but she still kept her house, cut her own grass, walked downtown to do errands and did church work. She gave up housekeeping at 95, when she suffered a bout of tendinitis from running up and down the steps to keep the basement dry during the groundwater flooding of 1993. Her mind remained sound until she entered a nursing home at 98. Then, in inactivity, she deteriorated quickly.

Muscle size and strength is important in sports: to avoid injury, to increase bone density, and to maintain heart health and physical attractiveness. But it is also supremely important to our whole body functioning and our day-to-day living.

Our body is an integrated system. A strong heart pumps blood out into our arteries at a high pressure (the top or systolic component of our blood pressure reading). But our muscles don't just use the blood, load it with carbon dioxide and other waste and send it back to the heart against gravity without providing their own push.

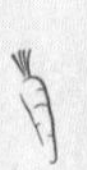

Our peripheral muscles too are pumps which provide the kick to send oxygen-depleted, waste-loaded blood back through the veins (the bottom or diastolic component of our blood pressure reading).

Our heart is the central pumping station, our peripheral muscles—all the way down to our hands and feet—are multiple substations that return the product in the pipeline.

Strong muscles are strong pumps on both ends of the system. They raise the rate at which our body uses its fuel. (No blood pressure medication can replace the kick a strong heart and strong peripheral muscles give blood transport. Medications correct some parts of the problems of low or high blood pressure, but muscle strength determines the whole system.)

CALORIES, WEIGHT, AND EXERCISE

The good news is that if we exercise, we live longer and the quality of our life is better. The bad news is that there's no stopping at any age without dire consequences. Ugh!

Clearly the only solution to this dilemma of exercise *ad infinitum* is to do things that you like to do that will tax you, but keep you injury free. How do we know what's what and what's enough?

Common sense goes a long way in evaluating activities. Obviously playing tennis expends more energy than playing baseball. Obviously, raking leaves takes more energy than planting a garden. Obviously, shoveling snow is more energy consumptive than washing windows. Obviously, running uses more energy than walking (except when you walk or run the same distance, then walking just takes more time).

Nevertheless, you need some scientifically established guidelines on weight and caloric intake and expenditure to figure out what is right just for you. That will take some time, some study, some figuring, and then, some discipline. But it will be just what you need: a plan established for you and your lifestyle.

You need a weight guide, although no general guide is a bible for you. Here is a generic guide. We like it because it adjusts for frame size. (All of these indices are available in various forms and complexities on the Internet.)

A body-mass index (BMI) table (pp. 24-25) also is helpful because it gives you a rough idea of body fat and can alert you to problems that may develop. Body Mass Index compares height to weight and assigns that comparative number. Too thin is as much concern as too fat, so take a look, knowing that the ideal is between 20 and 25.

In the nutrition chapters of this book, we stress that calories count, that the diet proponents who said that calories were not important were wrong. By moving away from calorie counting in the past 30 years, we have accumulated deadly weight gains. So we're recommending using our

HEIGHT AND WEIGHT TABLE – *MEN*

Height	Small frame	Med. frame	Large frame
5'2"	128-134	131-141	138-150
5'3"	130-136	133-143	140-153
5'4"	132-138	135-145	142-156
5'5"	134-140	137-148	144-160
5'6"	136-142	139-151	146-164
5'7"	138-145	142-154	149-168
5'8"	140-148	145-157	152-172
5'9"	142-151	148-160	155-176
5'10"	144-154	151-163	158-180
5'11"	146-157	154-166	161-184
6'	149-160	157-170	164-188
6'1"	152-164	160-174	168-192
6'2"	155-168	164-178	172-197
6'3"	158-172	167-182	176-202
6'4"	162-176	171-187	181-207

method (or one that is more tedious, but more accurate for you) to set a caloric intake for yourself.

(Health clubs and much standard exercise equipment measure the intensity of an effort in METs. A MET is the amount of oxygen consumed in one minute by a seated resting individual. If you run into METs, remember a MET and a calorie are roughly equivalent.)

Because we want you to establish an accurate guide that fits you to a T, we don't want to give a standard chart on how many calories you should consume a day. Follow our rough equivalents or buy or borrow some edition of Brian Sharkey's *Fitness and Health*—it's a wonderfully informative, easy-to-read general fitness guide.

HEIGHT AND WEIGHT TABLE — *WOMEN*

Height	Small frame	Med. frame	Large frame
4'10"	102-111	109-121	118-131
4'11"	103-113	111-123	120-134
5'	104-115	113-126	122-137
5'1"	106-118	115-129	125-140
5'2"	108-121	118-132	128-143
5'3"	111-124	121-135	131-147
5'4"	114-127	124-138	134-151
5'5"	117-130	127-141	137-155
5'6"	120-133	130-144	140-159
5'7"	123-136	133-147	143-163
5'8"	126-139	136-150	146-167
5'9"	129-142	139-153	149-170
5'10"	132-145	142-156	152-173
5'11"	135-148	145-159	155-176
6'	138-151	148-162	158-179

BODY MASS INDEX TABLE

BMI	19	20	21	22	23	24
Height	*Body Weight (lbs)*					
58"	91	96	100	105	110	115
59"	94	99	104	109	114	119
60"	97	102	107	112	118	123
61"	100	106	111	116	122	127
62"	104	109	115	120	126	131
63"	107	113	118	124	130	135
64"	110	116	122	128	134	140
65"	114	120	126	132	138	144
66"	118	124	130	136	142	148
67"	121	127	134	140	146	153
68"	125	131	138	144	151	158
69"	128	135	142	149	155	162
70"	132	139	146	153	161	167
71"	136	143	150	157	165	172
72"	140	147	154	162	169	177
73"	144	151	159	166	174	182
74"	148	155	163	171	179	186
75"	152	160	168	176	184	192
76"	156	164	172	180	189	197

25	26	27	28	29	30	31	32	33	34	35
Body Weight (lbs)										
119	124	129	134	138	143	148	153	158	162	167
124	128	133	138	143	148	153	158	163	168	173
128	133	138	143	148	153	158	163	168	174	179
132	137	143	148	153	158	164	169	174	180	185
136	142	147	153	158	164	169	175	180	186	191
141	146	152	158	163	169	175	180	186	191	197
145	151	157	163	169	174	180	186	192	197	204
150	156	162	168	174	180	186	192	198	204	210
155	161	167	173	179	186	192	198	204	210	216
159	166	172	178	185	191	198	204	211	217	223
164	171	177	184	190	197	203	210	216	223	230
169	176	182	189	196	203	209	216	223	230	236
174	181	188	195	202	209	216	222	229	236	243
179	186	193	200	208	215	222	229	236	243	250
184	191	199	206	213	221	228	235	242	250	258
189	197	204	212	219	227	235	242	250	257	265
194	202	210	218	225	233	241	249	256	264	272
200	208	216	224	232	240	248	256	264	272	279
205	213	221	230	238	246	254	263	271	279	287

To use the table, find the appropriate height in the left-hand column labeled Height. Move across to a given weight. The number at the top of the column is the BMI at that height and weight. Pounds have been rounded off.

MEASURING YOUR CALORIC EXPENDITURE

First establish your doing-nothing (basal) energy number: that is how many calories you would use in 24 hours of complete bedrest.

DOING-NOTHING ENERGY EXPENDITURE

Weight	**Expenditure** (24hrs)/calories
(Women)	
100 lb	1225 cal
120	1320
140	1400
160	1485
180	1575
(Men)	
140 lb	1550 cal
160	1640
180	1730
200	1815
220	1900

Second, adjust this basal number by multiplying it by a percentage based on what you do when you work:

Increase by

> 30% if you spend much of that eight hours sitting (whether that's at a computer, reading, or watching television);

> 40% if you do light activity (like office work, light housework, errand running, chauffeuring kids or stuff);

> 50% if you do more than light work;

> 60% if you do much more, but aren't moving 80% of the time;

- > 70% if you routinely do a moderate and steady amount of activity (like real housework or selling in which you are on your feet and moving);
- > 80% if you routinely walk, run, climb 80% of your workday (such as delivery work or heavy housework);
- > 90% or even 100% if you do heavy activity (such as construction, working on a receiving dock or other routine lifting and hauling).

Third, add those numbers and adjust the sum for age: subtracting 4% for every 10 years you are over 25.

Now you have a routine workday.

Time to figure in your recreational or nonwork activities. Calculate that by using our Chart A on page 28 (calories used in work and recreational activities) or Sharkey's similar, more complete chart. Multiply the calories used in your activities by the time you usually do them. Round out to represent a week; then divide by 7 to get a daily average. First use our Chart A for common work and recreational activities. (This scale assumes a weight of 150 pounds. If you weigh 125 decrease it by 1/6; if you weigh 175, increase it by 1/6 and so on.)

CHART A*

Activity	Cal/min
Driving a car	2.8
Walking indoors	3.2
Horseshoes	3.8
Housework	4.5
Baseball (not pitching)	4.7
Rowing (easy)	5.0
Golfing (walk)	5.0
Walking (3.5mph)	5.2
Gardening	5.6
Sawing with chainsaw	6.2
Canoeing (4mph)	7.0
Bowling (while active)	7.0
Snow shoveling	7.2
Walking down stairs	7.5
Walking up stairs	8.6
Volleyball (hard)	8.0
Basketball (hard)	9.0
Soccer (hard)	9.0
Tennis (hard)	10.
Handball/squash	10.
Mountain climbing	12.
Skipping rope	14
Judo/karate	14
Football (while active)	14.4
Cycling (hard)	15
Skating (hard)	15
Running (8 min mile)	15
Dancing (swing)	15.5
Skiing (racing/steep)	17.5
Swimming (easy-hard)	6.-17.5
Cross-country skiing	17.5
Running (6 min mile)	20
Running (5 min mile)	25

*Subtract 10% for weight under 150; add 10% for weight over 150.

Let's do calculations for Ed, 70; Tim, 36; and Dorothea, 71:

	Ed	**Tim**	**Dorothea**
Basal rate:	*1485*	*1400*	*1275*
Work Adjusted	+891(60%)	+840(60%)	+840(60%)
Age Adjust	-380(16%)	-90(4%)	-286(16%)
Activity Adjust	+1800	+1200	+390
	=3796	=3350	=1889

Clearly, if you are exercising at the rate that Ed and Tim do (as much as three hours a day), you have no trouble maintaining a competitive weight. They can eat almost anything, but neither eats junk food or fast food. Dorothea hasn't much room for those foods in 1900 calories. Contrary to either of the old folks, as a vegetarian and serious athlete, Tim has little trouble holding a long, lean frame. Ed struggles when he is not in strict training. It's a function of age and base metabolism.

All Ironman competitors are careful eaters. If they allow their weight to fluctuate more than 20% between serious training and off season, they are in serious trouble. Almost no professional athlete or serious contender eats fast food. It's just a fact of their life; no McDonald's, Wendy's, Hardees, Taco Bell, Long John Silver, KFC and the like. Even the chicken is heavy on calories and fat in comparison with its nutritional value.

Chapter 3

Aerobic Conditioning

INVENTING THE IRONMAN

The Hawaiian Ironman was dreamed up in 1977 by a group of macho military men. It was, of course, conceived in a bar. After arguing about which sport was more taxing, Navy Commander John Collins suggested they put Oahu's three endurance events (swim, bike, run) together, back to back.

The Waikiki Rough Water Swim was 2.4 miles, the Around-Oahu Bike Race was 112 and the Honolulu Marathon was, of course, 26.2. Collins reportedly said, "Whoever finishes it first, we'll call the Iron Man." The feat seemed impossible.

That was what intrigued them and challenged them. It was a dare, a test of their machismo. They set a date and recruited a few friends—very few. On February 18, 1978, on Oahu they set up a course. The entry fee was $3. Fifteen men started.

Twelve finished. Their times are a joke. None would qualify for a competitive spot in today's races. They did not invent the sport (that was done in San Diego in 1974); but they put it to the test it celebrates today.

That doesn't, however, stand as today's ultimate endurance test. There are double Ironman competitions and even triple ones. People enter; people do it; people walk away, rather than drop dead.

Training methods differ. One winner swears by sprints and speed workouts that postpone fatigue a few minutes more each time. Another values the long, slow workouts that stress the muscles to endure and grow constantly stronger. No one who stands on the podium the night after the race to receive a trophy has forgone either element in training: speed or endurance.

Perhaps there really is no limit to the kinds of stress and endurance the tried and trained human body is capable of. Today some 1500 competitors participate in the Hawaii race; to do so 34,000 of them take part in Ironman and half-Ironman qualifying races throughout the world.

No one does it without training. That is the Ironman's ultimate secret. He or she has challenged his or her body in the months—and probably years—prior to the race, constantly, but gradually, demanding more and the body responds with more.

The human body is a totally integrated system. It is, says Ed, no stronger than its weakest link. Its systems—muscular/skeletal, respiratory, digestive, circulatory, nervous, endocrine and so on—all contribute to the effort. Each must do its job better or the whole breaks down.

That strengthening doesn't happen in a day, a week, a month. But put under stress, each system responds.

ENERGY FOR MOVEMENT

Within our muscles are two distinct fibers and two distinct systems that produce energy to move muscles. Our fast-twitch fiber uses *anaerobic* (without oxygen) energy. It uses the chemical ATP (adenosine triphosphate) already stored in the muscle to respond immediately to demand, but that energy lasts just a few seconds. Besides the stored ATP, muscles also contain glycogen (the storage form of glucose) that fast-twitch fibers can convert anaerobically to more ATP; but that source too is limited and can last no more than three minutes.

A sprinter running a dash calls on this energy source; so does a deer startled in the woods or an antelope on the

Serengeti. We assume that in evolution this system developed for survival.

Since anaerobic energy depends on finite stored sources—and since converting glycogen to energy produces waste (chiefly lactic acid)—anaerobic energy can't be sustained. Fuel runs out; waste builds up; muscle fatigues.

Then slow-twitch fiber using *aerobic* energy takes over. It produces ATP from oxygen delivered to the muscles by the blood. This delivery system also is a waste disposal system that carries away the harmful byproducts of ATP production.

Probably training can't change the ratio of fast-twitch to slow-twitch fibers you are born with. Sprinters are sprinters because they have more fast twitch fibers and marathoners are marathoners because they have fewer. But clearly training can change the efficiency of the aerobic system. With training, muscles produce more ATP and become better at disposing of waste and postponing fatigue. They do so because with training, the muscle's blood supply increases dramatically.

Our muscles need nutrition, as well as oxygen, but they draw that from any number of sources stored within the body. Fat is the most efficient storage method.

DELIVERING OXYGEN

By making intense demands on the body, Ironman competitors strain the respiratory and circulatory systems. Their muscles need more oxygen and their body responds by revving up its systems to deliver it.

At rest, we breathe about 15 times a minute. About 250 ml of oxygen enters the blood each minute and 200 ml of carbon dioxide leaves it. This blood/gas exchange takes place in the hundreds of millions of alveoli of our lungs. (Spread out flat—if that were possible—our lung surface would cover about half a tennis court.)

One of the obvious effects of exercise is that we breathe harder. We huff and puff to get more oxygen; we do this by creating more space for the lungs to expand. During our normal activity, expiration is a passive movement. During heavy exercise, the muscles that control our diaphragm pull the ribs down, creating a greater pressure drop in the chest cavity. With that expanded space to fill, more air rushes into our lungs. When we do this enough, our respirator muscles grow stronger to make it easier to breathe deeper.

Exercise improves our ventilation overall. It not only brings in more oxygen, it carries out more carbon dioxide and other waste. In one experiment, the respiratory endurance of healthy adult men and women improved as much as 16% in 20 weeks of running.

At first, we breathe deeper without breathing faster. Through training, we can increase the amount of air we take in with each breath by 50%. Then, as exercise becomes more intense and demand for oxygen increases further, athletes increase their breathing rate. Between the two, we can dramatically increase the amount of oxygen delivered and waste removed.

Breathing deeper simply increases the efficiency of our lungs. We use portions of our lungs that normally remain unused, which is very good. That first causes muscle fatigue because we are using muscles we do not ordinarily use, and then, of course, muscles grow and strengthen.

In addition, the respiratory system is so closely tied to our cardiovascular system, improving one inevitably benefits the other.

Aerobic training improves: respiratory efficiency, blood volume, distribution and delivery of blood to muscles, stroke volume (the amount of blood put out by the heart in one beat) and cardiac output (CO—the heart's total output in one minute). About half of these benefits are respiratory and half are circulatory.

Our heart—a beating, pulsating, thrusting muscle—sits in the center of a life-sustaining double loop that is our cardiovascular system: heart, arteries, veins, lungs. It sends blood through its 60,000 miles of tubing 1440 times a day, 43,800 times a month, 525,600 times a year—to carry nourishment to and waste from every tissue.

The heart, like every other tissue, responds to demand. At rest, its demand for oxygen and nutrition is low. In light exercise it can increase eight to 12 times. In strenuous exercise (or dire emergency) it can increase 20 times.

Our CO (the amount of blood pumped by the heart each minute) determines how our body meets these demands. It depends on two factors: the amount of blood ejected with each beat (stroke volume) and rate of beat. The ejection capacity depends directly on the strength of the heart muscle.

Increasing demand systematically through exercise directly increases the heart's capacity. Although that is determined to some extent by the activity or passivity of our youth, it can always be improved, even for those who have heart problems. However, always be cautious. If you have a history of heart problems, personal or family, have a stress test before attempting strenuous exercise of any kind. Then, for everyone, begin slowly. Listen to your body for feedback and never attempt to power through prolonged pain.

Building heart muscle is a long, slow—but sure—process that every Ironman competitor has gone through and mastered. His or her training goals have been to extend the volume of blood ejected with each beat by increasing the heart's ability to contract and, by this strength, to slow the time it takes to reach maximal heart rate.

The moderate exerciser achieves the same goals, but to a more moderate extent. The moderate exerciser will know he/she is extending aerobic capacity because speed and endurance will increase steadily and his/her pulse rate may drop slightly. That is probably enough. For the endurance athlete, monitoring progress with a heart monitor is essential.

Since he began endurance training 20 years ago, Ed has driven his resting heart rate from 70 to 45. Now, his heart is so strong and its stroke volume so high that raising his beat requires more and more physical stress. His maximum capacity is about 155 beats a minute. That's the heady rate of elite endurance athletes whether they are triathletes, basketball or hockey players, scullers or distance runners and swimmers.

Chapter 4

Right Direction Wrong Road

In the United States we suffer from plenty. There are grim statistics about overweight and obesity. One fact alone is telling: 75% of our ailments come from poor diet and sedentary lifestyle. We need to take the matter of our weight, our health and our lifestyle into our own hands and do something about it. No one else can. Since we were told to exercise, we have. Multimillion dollar industries have grown up around keeping fit. Fifty years ago, only kids, prizefighters, and bodybuilders used gyms. Now there are far more gyms on U.S. street corners than ice cream parlors.

We have had successes. In the past 40 years, the average American consumption of fat has dropped from 44% to 34% The average consumption of refined sugar has dropped and the number of adults over 25 who smoke has fallen precipitously. Despite the alarming spread of smoking among children and teenagers, fewer North Americans smoke than in almost any other industrialized nation.

The jogging craze began at the University of Oregon in Eugene in the 1950s. It has done us worlds of good, although overall the number of Americans who exercise regularly has reached a plateau.

In 1996 the Boston Marathon marked its centennial, but 50 years ago it was one of the few places to run a marathon. Now two million Americans run marathons in cities and towns from Portland, Oregon (where hundreds also *walk* the marathon), to Portland, Maine, from San Diego to Sarasota. The Ironman now draws 30,000 participants a year to grueling *qualifying* competitions.

Three things have gone wrong to make us grow fatter and less healthy because of it:

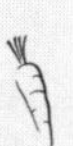

Don't believe for one second that America will not solve its problem of poor health and fitness. We will; you will. But we needed to be better informed and today we can be.

> We want a quick fix. We are so wealthy, why shouldn't we have the best, and the best is the easiest thing that works.

> We are so anxious that we're easily mislead by well-meaning "experts" offering an easy way—often selling things from books to pills.

> We're too willing to turn responsibility over to someone else. It won't work. The only person who can decide to make you healthy is you.

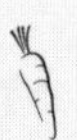

To be healthy we need to eat right and exercise. That is absolutely all there is to it. Don't worry about reducing stress; that will come.

The next chapters are about eating right and diets. You need to understand which fuels your body needs and how to feed it for efficient performance.

In the past half century, obesity has risen by 50%. A recent study found that 63% of American men 25 years and older and 55% of women are overweight. Obesity, as measured by the body-mass index that compares weight to height, now stands at 18%; in 1993 it was 12%. Alarmingly, one of every five children is now overweight (the figure has doubled in 20 years).

There are wonderful, breakthrough nutrition and diet plans

out there. You may have read and followed a half dozen of them. But very simply, a diet plan that works for someone else may not work for you. You need to plan along simple guidelines that fit your lifestyle. If your plan doesn't; it won't work.

Sadly, in the past the people responsible for public health haven't always done a good job. For many years, there was no nutritional information on the food we bought to bring home or the food we ate out. Now, the nutritional information printed on nearly all grocery-store foods is a godsend. It tells us all we need to know for healthful eating. Use it.

And there are dozens of books and booklets that give the same healthful analysis of the foods offered by fast-food restaurants.

Still, not all "guides" are sufficient in themselves. You need to be an informed consumer. That is what this section aims to make you.

As an example, let's look at the U.S. Department of Agriculture's recent dietary guideline: the food pyramid which comes into our homes on the back of foods that would convince us of their healthfulness.

Does it help? Yes, somewhat, if we know enough to refine it.

Should we eat 6-11 servings of grains a day? Yes, if we eat stone-ground wheat bread; brown rice; whole-grain cereal; and other close-to-whole, close-to-unprocessed grains. No, if we eat puffed up, sweetened, processed cereals; doughnuts; bagels (yes, bagels), and egg noodles and pastas in butter and cream.

Do we need 2-3 servings of meat, poultry, fish, dry beans, eggs, and nuts a day? Perhaps, if those are grilled salmon; no-fat refried beans; breast of turkey; egg-white omelets. No, if we eat a thick beef filet; a bacon/cheeseburger (with or without bun); fried eggs and sausage; barbecued ribs and fried fish.

Should we eat 5-9 servings of fruits and vegetables? Yes, under almost any circumstances. Yet these need careful selection. French-fries, baked potatoes (with or without butter or sour cream) or frozen potato puffs; buttered cooked carrots; candied sweet potatoes; salt-pork flavored greens; papayas, mangoes, avocados or bananas and frozen juices are not the best choices (the juices have the fruit fiber processed out).

Do we need to use fats, oils and sweets sparingly? Yes, but there are essential fatty acids that we don't make in our body, so using the right oils sparingly is necessary.

Is the USDA food pyramid dangerous to our health? Yes, if we remain uneducated about nutrition. But it is never too late to learn. At present too many of us are eating ourselves into the grave.

First and foremost, no diet works for everyone and, equally important, no diet alone works. We need to exercise. To lose weight, we have to use more calories than we take in. To maintain weight, we need to make that an even exchange.

The secret to a healthy lifestyle: EXERCISE—run, walk, dance, play sports, bicycle, swim, chase children or grandchildren, garden, rake leaves, walk the steps. Your body was meant to be used as long as you have the breath to use it. Too frequently we mothball it after we reach 40.

Finally, fall off the wagon every once in a while. It's what Freud called "regression in service to the ego." Simple concept: regress so that you relax a little and feel good about yourself.

If you are going to do these things, what do you need to know?

You need to know basically what these chapters are going to tell you. There are beautiful books from knowledgeable authorities available. Buy or borrow at least one. Remember, always consider the source.

Your body is an elegant machine. It wants hard work and sufficient—not abundant—nutrition.

MEMORIZE AND LIVE WITH FIVE GUIDELINES:

> **Give up diets—all of them and their trappings: pills, gadgets, surgeries, bars, drinks, herbs, wraps, zones, factors, supplements, everything. Never believe another diet proponent unless you know that this plan will help you achieve a short-term goal (like original weight loss or weight loss to meet a training goal).**

> **Exercise, at least moderately, both aerobically (running, walking, tennis, blading) and with strength training (free weights or machines).**

> **Eat less and eat as naturally as possible.**

> **Practice balance: in exercise, stress reduction (which will come naturally if you do the first three) and nutrition.**

> **Don't be fickle. Find a way of eating, working, relaxing that keeps you slim, trim, and healthy. Then stick to it through hell and high water; stress and relaxation; weekdays, workdays, and not-at-home days.**

NECESSARY FUELS

Our body requires three fuels: oxygen, food, and water. Over a period of time, it must take in all three, process each, and send the energy produced from brain to heel in a never-ending stream. A steady supply of oxygen is the most critical. Aside from the very limited capacity of our lungs and blood, we have no oxygen stores.

Oxygenation takes place every second of every minute. All fish, fowl, amphibians, and mammals—including humans—have systems for drawing oxygen from air or water. Strangely, none of these systems has a backup.

Nutritionally, we need to look critically at our oxygen supply because within the past century it has changed: it has become enormously polluted and poses new danger to our good health. Those dangers are from biological particulates identified as *free radicals* that are made within our body. Our body's natural defenses against these are substances called *antioxidants.*

FREE RADICALS, ANTIOXIDANTS AND AGING

For exercisers, understanding free radicals and antioxidants is terribly important. The more we breathe our polluted air, the greater our danger of free radical damage and our need of antioxidants.

One of the two major theories of aging attributes the process to the accumulated damage caused by free radicals. The second is a program theory. They are not mutually exclusive. In fact, the more we learn, the surer we are that disease and death result from some combination of the two.

The program theory says that we age because we are programmed to do so. The damage theory is that free radicals cause damage that is eventually irreversible.

Clearly, aging and death are part of a natural process to improve the species. For survival, nature clears out the old to make room for younger members who are better able to contribute to the overall health of the species.

We know that in humans and other animals, some cells eventually enter a state where they cannot replicate. Geneticists have uncovered molecular clocks that govern what is known as *replicative senescence.* When this state is reached and no new cells can be born, the cell dies. It is likely then that we are programmed to age and die.

Yet science currently tells us that man's natural life span is between 115 and 120 years. If we don't achieve that something has gone wrong. We've been the victims of our lifestyle or environment, natural or man-made disasters, heredity, change, or combinations of these. Several of these factors do irreparable damage through the rampages of free radicals.

As our body converts inhaled oxygen to water, it creates some free radicals (and other substances in the category of *active oxygen species.*) These are molecules with an unpaired electron capable of independent existence. Their electron needs a mate and they scavenge for it from whatever they come in contact with. In doing so, they damage the substances they have stolen an electron from.

If free radicals are so dangerous, why does our body tolerate this?

Because some free radicals perform work—destructive work—that needs to be done to defend the body. Some kill cancer cells. Some effect the process of cell suicide that defends against the spread of irradiation, drug toxicity, viral infections. Free radicals are part of the body's immune system. We need them and we produce them naturally from within.

However, within the past 150 years, man-made pollution in the form of harmful toxins in the air has introduced enormous new dangers from free radicals. As we breathe in soot, smog, industrial waste, auto exhaust, we take in these toxins. Smoking and chewing tobacco introduce toxins that eventually pass into our bloodstream. In addition, we ingest toxins with the foods we eat and the water we drink. Overall we are in much greater danger from free radical airborne toxins than we were before the Industrial Revolution.

Our body knew it needed to keep free radicals in check, so it developed defenses: *antioxidants.* These prevent free radicals from being formed, trap them once they have formed or repair the damage they cause. Amazing!

Today we know that most of the chronic and degenerative diseases of aging originate in free radical damage. (In 1999 Dr. Lester Packer of the University of California, Berkeley—

the leading researcher in this field—wrote an excellent booklet entitled *The Antioxidant Network and Healthy Aging.* Published by Infoceuticals, Inc., which under the registered trademark of Cyberpac, Inc., sells antioxidant supplements, this booklet argues clearly and succinctly for the damage theory of aging. Dr. Packer recommends taking supplements that contain what he calls an antioxidant network of vitamins and minerals.)

An alternative to supplementation is to consume a diet rich in antioxidants—vitamins such as B complex, C, E, beta carotene; minerals: selenium, zinc, copper, manganese, iron; ascorbic acid, and BHT(butylated hydroxytoluenel), to name a few. Such a diet is not hard to build. It would be based on eating large amounts of fresh fruits and vegetables and drinking green tea.

The body's first line of defense is a group of enzymes that scavenge for free radicals and destroy them before they can do harm. These enzymes need the minerals zinc, copper, selenium, manganese, and iron to work efficiently. If we once had an adequate supply of these, that supply has been overcome by the increase in toxins we currently take into our body.

The body's second line of defense is a group of vitamins—chiefly, B complex, C, E, and beta carotene—that quench the action of the free radicals and help repair the damage they do.

For serious athletes, dietary supplementation may be necessary because athletes greedily breathe the air of civilization. If we could train in pure air we would be better off, but we can't.

However, despite the increased danger from training, leading an active life through exercise is still far better than being sedentary. No one—absolutely no one—doubts that the benefits of exercise far outweigh the increased risks.

BACK TO BASIC NUTRITION

Unlike oxygen, fresh water and food are efficiently stored in the body, so that supplies of each can be occasional. Our capacity to store water is limited; our capacity to store nutrients is not.

That capacity is great and highly refined. It has been our salvation for eons. Only in the past few thousand years have humans had a steady supply of food for nutrition. Before, we often had to live off our stored fat. (And that is what diets aim to do.) Now, however, in most of the world, food supply has far outstripped the energy needed to obtain it. And we grow fat.

Chapter 5

Eating Right

THE MACRONUTRIENTS

Our basic nutritional needs are macronutrients: carbohydrates, fats, and protein. These provide energy and help maintain and repair the body.

Fiber is sometimes listed as a macronutrient. Strictly speaking, it isn't a nutrient at all, since it never burns to produce energy. But we now see that fiber is so essential to a healthy diet, that grouping it with the basic components makes some sense.

Carbohydrates are the base of any nutritional pyramid. They are the main fuel burned for energy. However, all carbohydrates are not alike; some are complex; some are simple. Complex carbohydrates—those that come from whole, unprocessed grains and vegetables—should make up more than half of our daily diet.

Simple carbohydrates—actually, the sugars: fructose, glucose (also called dextrose), lactose, and sucrose and the like—should make up no more than 10% of our daily carbohydrate intake.

Though the body breaks down almost all carbohydrates into glucose—the simple sugar that is carried by the blood to cells for energy—the differentiation of carbohydrates is essential. Most complex carbohydrates carry with them large amounts of fiber, and because of this, they metabolize far more slowly than the simple sugars.

Being ignorant of the difference between simple and complex carbohydrates has caused America to grow increasingly fat.

Basically, simple carbohydrates turn into stored fat. They metabolize quickly, raising our blood sugar in a surge. The pancreas rushes in much insulin. That tells the liver it has excess glucose. So the liver does what it is supposed to do with excesses. It converts them to fat for storage.

Complex carbohydrates enter the blood more gradually. There is no rush of insulin and no storage signal. The body uses the glucose to produce energy now.

Thus the kind of carbohydrates we consume (as well as how many) determines how much of the potential energy our body stores as fat.

For the past 40 years, health officials have told us to cut fat, and we have. We have drastically (and wisely) decreased meat intake. But, after that we went wrong.

Experts told us to use carbohydrates to replace the fat we were losing and add the bulk that would make us feel full and satisfied. That advice is deadly, however, without two caveats:

> watch your caloric intake

> monitor the kind of carbohydrates

If we had really eaten more plain fruits and vegetables, that would have done it—but we haven't. We've loaded our vegetables with butter and sour cream, our salads with dressings, and our breads and pastas with butter and cream sauces, and sometimes we deep fried it all.

Fiber provides the grist that makes the body's mill work efficiently and smoothly. It's broken down into soluble fiber, which dissolves in water, and insoluble fiber, which does not. Those distinctions, however, are not terribly meaningful.

What all fiber has in common is that it cannot be

digested by enzymes in the human intestinal tract. It moves along in its stringy forms as waste sweeping the smooth muscle inside the stomach and intestines as it moves. It also provides adequate bulk to allow the body to reduce the amount of water in waste without making that waste hard.

The benefits of a high-fiber diet are hard to assess because fiber is never taken in isolation. It's a part of foods that tend to be low in fat and protein and high in antioxidants and trace vitamins and minerals. However, studies indicate that a high-fiber diet lessens the risks of an infamous roll-call of diseases: colon and rectal cancer, heart disease, diabetes, obesity, breast cancer, and a slew of intestinal ailments.

THE MICRONUTRIENTS

The second essential element of the human diet is micronutrients—the vitamins and minerals—present and needed in very small amounts. Micronutrients generally do not provide energy. They regulate body chemistry and help repair and build tissue.

Vitamins, a relative newcomer to scientific vocabulary, are organic substances that regulate functions within cells. With the exception of vitamins D and K, our body makes every vitamin we need. We now believe that our body needs 13 vitamins: A, C, D, E, K, and eight B vitamins—thiamine, riboflavin, niacin, pantothenic acid, B-6, B-12, folacin, and biotin. We convert beta carotene to vitamin A, but beta carotene also seems to have a separate role as an antioxidant.

Vitamins are fat-soluble (A,D,E, and K) or water-soluble (the B vitamins and C). The body generally stores fat-soluble vitamins for long periods (usually in the liver or fat tissue). The water-soluble vitamins are stored for only short periods. They need to be replenished frequently.

Unfortunately, the water-soluble vitamins are those that are damaged by cooking, so our diets need to be full of sources of the B vitamins and C that can be eaten raw or with the water they are cooked in. Fortunately, the whole grains we eat as cereals and starches (rice, barley, oats, couscous, bulgur wheat) are rich in several B vitamins and dairy products contain others. Even more fortunately, a whole list of the fruits we eat raw are plentiful sources of C.

Unfortunately, a few vitamins taken in mega doses are toxic. This kind of overdose is rare and can't really happen naturally, but it warns that not all supplementation is helpful. Take care.

WATER

Water is the third essential element in the human diet. It is a basic component of all foods. It provides the fluid medium for all body chemistry, blood circulation, and removal of waste. It also plays an important role in maintaining body temperature.

It's important to remember that water is such an essential element that our body has learned to hoard it and recycle it. The body removes as much water as it can before elimination. We need enormous amounts of water and diets that drop the body's water—as many do—are dangerous in the long run.

Although water is essential, remember that drinking fluid is not the total answer to rehydration. Besides drinking water, eat foods that contain both water and certain trace minerals that increase its absorption. (The sports drinks were developed to increase absorption by supplying some trace minerals.)

How much drinking bottled water helps depends, of course, on both its source and its purification. First, you should know what is missing *and* what is added in your public water and what is added and subtracted from your bottled substitute. There are standards set and many of the bottled waters adhere to these and display their certification.

Perhaps the greatest advantage of bottled water isn't its content but its portability. Having water handy makes people drink more water and that is very good, but it might be just as good if the water inside the bottle came from the tap. Your choice and the quality of your public water will be determinants here.

Call your city health department to find out your water source, how it is purified, and what is added for that purpose and for public health. Most departments can send an analysis of public water and a comparison with other U.S. communities. Use that information to decide if you want to drink from the tap, use bottled water, or use additional purification.

All food contains water—think of the noticeable amounts in zucchini, cucumbers, tomatoes, watermelon. If we eat foods raw, we ingest the water and with it the vitamins and trace minerals it contains. The minute we process foods—most notably by cooking, but also by pulverizing or salting—we diminish the water and its health-building components.

Eating fruits and vegetables raw (and with their skins, if possible) is the best way to get their full nutritive value. Next best is to eat them with the water they have been cooked in. Third best is to use as little additional water as necessary in cooking to retain the water-soluble vitamins—again the B vitamins and C.

HOW WE USE THE MACRONUTRIENTS

Our body constantly burns a mixture of macronutrients for energy. Carbohydrates are the most efficient fuel because they break down quickly to produce energy quickly. That, of course, is how we come to believe that a glass of orange juice or a candy bar is an efficient way to produce energy quickly.

In terms of body-efficiency, however, the price of that energy is very high. The sugars—natural or processed—are quickly absorbed into the bloodstream and trigger a massive insulin release which, in turn, has the terrible results we described simply early in this chapter.

At rest and at low levels of activity, half of the body's energy is produced by burning carbohydrates.

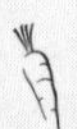

Fat, either from food or body stores, provides energy, but less quickly than carbohydrates. When our muscles' need for energy has been sustained for 20 or 30 minutes, our body begins to burn more fat than carbohydrate. The longer you tax the muscle through exercise, and/or the longer you go without resupply (food or drink) the more body fat is burned for fuel.

Thirty years ago in *Fit or Fat,* Covert Bailey warned against restricting calories—mainly carbohydrates—without exercise. Given self-induced famine, the body responds by consuming itself. That's just what we want it to do when we want to lose weight. However, being very wise, our body first consumes tissue that it isn't using.

After a few days of a severe diet, it says, in effect, "Wow, I'm not getting enough fuel here. I'll have to tap my storehouse. Well, fat is my most efficient storehouse, so I maybe shouldn't get rid of too much of it. Maybe I can find a source that's not essential to my well being right now."

If you are not exercising, that tissue is muscle. So the body uses both fat and muscle to sustain itself. If you reduce intake without exercise, you will end up with more fat and less muscle than you had before you began.

Finally, the nutritional information we have heard for years has not all stood the test of time. For instance, not all cholesterol is alike and not all clogs our arteries. On the cholesterol front, eggs are not the bad eggs they were once said to be. Not all carbohydrates are good for you; not all fats are bad. Consult a good nutritional guide and read labels. Both are essential to building a healthy diet.

Chapter 6

About Diets

There are seldom fewer than three diet books on the *New York Times* list of the best selling works of nonfiction. How sad!

We try on diets more often than we change our bed sheets but with little result.

To separate the good from the bad, let's try to understand how the major diets work. You may want to fit their strengths and weaknesses to your body and lifestyle. You may use them to meet a specific short-term goal such as initial weight loss.

If you haven't gotten the message that no diet works without exercise, we haven't said it often enough, clearly enough.

That is a fundamental message of this book.

In review we'll use generic terms:

> Diets that restrict carbohydrates and load protein;

> High-protein diets that don't restrict carbohydrates;

> Diets that severely restrict caloric intake;

> Diets that severely cut fat intake;

> Diets that are chiefly concerned with insulin production;

> Diets that are chiefly concerned with food combinations and other somewhat quirky assumptions.

HIGH PROTEIN, LOW CARBOHYDRATE DIET

These diets work. They eat body fat and people lose weight. People feel better about themselves and generally are healthier because they are not carrying all the weight that strains the heart and almost every other body system.

These diets seldom restrict calories; you eat as much as you want of anything but carbohydrates. However, because meat consumption is high, these diets do little to reduce—and may even elevate—blood-level cholesterol.

These diets basically starve the body of carbohydrates. The body's chief nutrient *is* carbohydrates. If you don't give it enough or you give it carbohydrates so seldom that it can't sustain itself on them, it turns to stored nutrient sources: fat.

These diets supply sufficient calories so that the body doesn't turn muscle into food. It lives off stored fat (the process is *ketosis* because it produces substances called ketones which build up in the blood).

But these diets are not natural. The excess protein strains the kidney. Excess ketones may cause nausea, dehydration, lightheadedness, and abnormal heart rhythms. Ketosis is not a normal body state long-term. It occurs when fatty acids don't completely oxidize because of the carbohydrate deficiency. It is observed in starvation and diabetes.

However these diets have worked well for millions of people for years—they were first proposed in the 1860s and have enjoyed resurgence periodically. In recent years, no scientific studies have been published in any peer-review medical journal that prove these diets sound and healthy. On the other hand, people on these diets haven't succumbed en masse to kidney exhaustion or any other fatal or debilitating ailment. But then, perhaps few people have strictly followed any version of them for as long as 10 or 20 years.

All science says that these diets cannot be healthy in the long run.

The Atkins diet—the current best-seller proponent—fits America's love of meat, cheese, and dairy consumption so well, it is the easiest diet in America to get on, lose fat, lose pounds, and even stay on.

Other versions of the severely restricted carbohydrate diets exist. One limits carbohydrates by cutting them from its dieters' intake 23 hours a day. Dieters eat anything and in any amount once a day and eat no-carbohydrates any other time. Scientifically, it works basically the same as the Atkins plan.

HIGH PROTEIN DIETS THAT DO NOT SEVERELY RESTRICT CARBOHYDRATES

Many of the cautions of the previous high-protein diets apply here also, except these plans do not rely on ketosis.

The average American takes in about 12% to 15% of his /her daily calories in protein. Most of these diets raise that level to at least 30% by increasing the dieter's consumption of meats (muscle) or soy products and extracts.

If our body made muscle from muscle, that would make sense; but it doesn't. It breaks all protein down to its constituent amino acids and circulates those acids through the bloodstream. There are hundreds of proteins used by the body and each is different. Each process that needs certain proteins builds its specific proteins from the component parts circulating in the blood.

Excess protein overworks the kidneys and the liver, leaches calcium and phosphorus from bones, and increases the danger of kidney stones. Many of these reactions are the body's attempt to keep its normal pH balance. Animal products are acidic; plant foods are alkaline.

If our increased protein comes from meat, eggs, cheeses, and other dairy products—and it usually does, even if the diet calls for some increased plant proteins—acid intake overcomes alkalai intake. The body searches for neutralizers somewhere within. It finds alkaline calcium and phosphorus in bones and leaches alkalai from that source. The Nurses Health Study found that women who took in 95 grams of protein a day, compared to those who took in only 68 grams, had a 22% greater risk of forearm fractures.

In addition, by stressing protein intake, these diets often raise blood-level cholesterol dangerously high. This results in all of the increased risks of heart disease and cancers that we've been warned about for 50 years.

There is no sound scientific evidence to prove that high protein diets (diets that in effect replace carbohydrates with protein) result in sound weight loss. They do initially, however, shed body water and thereby pounds, so they seem to work quickly and almost magically. But there is no magic and there is long-range potential for real harm.

DIETS THAT SEVERELY LIMIT CALORIC INTAKE

These diets starve the body to induce it to consume stored energy supplies and thus produce weight loss. They come in various degrees of severity measured in calorie restrictions. The most severe restrict a woman's caloric consumption to 800 calories a day. The less severe set that goal at 1000 to 1200 calories.

In the second chapter, we hedged on giving healthful caloric-intake numbers. We suggested there a formula to figure your needs as an individual. For the purpose of comparison here, however, we use the following. A woman who exercises moderately needs between 1500 and 2000 calories a day to provide the necessary nutrients and fiber and to balance intake and use. For men that range is from 2200 to 2700. The primary object of restricting calories to far below those ranges is to induce the body to used stored fat for energy. Often, however, the result is a loss of water and muscle as well.

All 800 calorie or less diets need to be monitored by a doctor and a nutritionist. Without careful guidance these diets can be extremely dangerous. In addition, to supply the essential nutrients, many of these rely on high-priced supplements. They may be beneficial under unusual circumstances, but normally no one needs to starve the body to that extent for that kind of quick weight loss. Simply don't, unless you are grossly obese and your doctor recommends and monitors your plan. Otherwise, plan ahead to reduce weight more gradually.

A score of other diet plans limit calories to 1000 to 1200 a day. The most common use liquid diet drinks and supplements of 200/250 calories to replace two meals a day. They urge dieters then to eat a third meal rich in fruits, vegetables and protein, but caution that this meal must not exceed 600 calories. Since the diet drinks—either liquid or powder added to skim milk—are fortified with vitamins, minerals and some fat, they are both nutritionally sound and temporarily satisfying. And they are both convenient and generally inexpensive.

The downside of any diet that uses supplements to restrict calories is that it doesn't teach healthy eating habits and a return to normal food can be disastrous. In addition, we know too little about the body's chemical reactions to rely heavily on chemical fortifications to replace natural plant foods.

Crash dieting, no matter what form it takes, usually doesn't work in the long run. Studies show that laboratory animals lose more weight faster the first time an extreme calorie-restricted diet is used, but effectiveness diminishes with every repeat and weight comes back faster.

Low calorie diets also increase the risk of blood pressure problems and coronary heart disease because they interfere with the body's natural metabolism. In addition, if they don't succeed as promised, they're psychologically harmful and stressful. They indicate that you can't succeed where millions of others have. Nonsense.

If you starve the body and do not exercise, your body will not only consume its fat, but its muscle. Muscle weighs more than fat, so the diets seem to be succeeding wonderfully, but they are not. Without exercising, any restriction of calories to less than 1200 a day may make you slimmer, but you will not be fit.

A major failure of diets that call for less than 1000 calories a day, however, is that they are so unnatural they cannot be maintained. Few humans can starve voluntarily for long.

That brings us to a final drawback to starvation diets. They can induce eating disorders, particularly in young women. There is growing concern among coaches, trainers and parents of young women athletes that slim and sleek has crossed from healthy to dangerous and needs to be rethought. The same rethinking needs to apply to the emphasis we place on skinny being beautiful and desirable. It can drive young women to anorexia and bulimia.

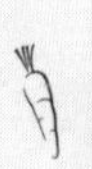

Remember, the body is nothing more than a biochemical machine. Its basic arithmetic is caloric intake/output. Eat more than you use and you will gain weight; eat less than you expend and you will lose weight.

The key to successful, long-term weight loss is to use more calories through exercise and take in fewer, but to make the calories consumed supply nutrition. Obviously, the key to weight maintenance is the same. Any food that contains calories (including alcohol) but does not proportionally supply nutrition is a junk food.

DIETS THAT SEVERELY LIMIT FAT INTAKE

There are three issues that overlap here. The first deals with diets that severely limit fat. Another deals with the question of what fat limitation makes the most effective American diet. A third looks at the disastrous results that have followed America's blind fetish with fat reduction.

Dr. Dean Ornish has for years advocated a diet of 10% fat. He began his program to demonstrate that such a diet—combined with exercise and stress-reduction techniques—was as effective as surgery in combating heart disease. Unlike many other diet gurus, Ornish has carefully documented his claims with replicable scientific studies. The science behind his intervention is unquestionable.

Shortly after the success of his first book—*Reversing Heart Disease*—he published a second, still aimed at heart patients, but somewhat widening the use of his plan. He has continued to widen his plan so that he advocates its use by anyone who wants and needs to control his or her weight. Despite his contention, however, it is most successful for those to whom weight control is essential.

One common complaint about low-fat diets is that they leave the dieter feeling hungry. It's true. Fats digest more slowly than carbohydrates because the body needs to break them down into tiny droplets. Because they stay in the stomach longer, they promote a feeling of well being. Too little fat in a diet leaves a dieter perpetually unsatisfied.

Many proponents of extremely low-fat diets are responsible scientists and nutritionists. Their diets stress the importance of eating fruits and vegetables for their complex carbohydrates. Some include supplements of omega 3 oils to ensure adequate essential fatty acids. Most are sound and produce healthy weight loss for those who follow the diets religiously.

Ornish argues that his "is a diet that many people can follow in the real world.... Big changes are often easier than small ones because most people feel so much better, so quickly, that it reframes the reason for change from fear of dying to joy of living."

Would that that were true for the average American. Statistics say it isn't. Studies from the University of Washington in Seattle indicate that reducing total fat to 30% and reducing saturated fat to from 7 to 8% of that total was as effective in lowering blood-level cholesterol as diets with less total fat. These studies further indicate that participants had no difficulty sticking to the 30% level, but that Americans have a great deal of trouble with a more stringent fat-reduction diet.

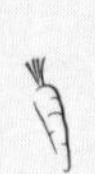

The American Heart Association recommends that heart patients consume no more than 30% of their daily calories from fat and limit saturated fat to 10% of that total. As a nation, we are nearly there. From 1960 to 1999 we reduced fat intake from 44% to 34%. Yet many of us have, in that same time, become dangerously overweight and 18% of us are obese.

Our fixation on fat reduction lets us bypass other important issues. We focused on fat and ignored the difference between simple and complex carbohydrates and, more recently, the glycemic index. In addition, we didn't watch our calories. We thought that if a food was no fat or low fat, we could eat as much of it as we wanted.

Many of the foods we ate instead of fat—white breads, standard "wheat" breads, other refined flour products (even bagels and crackers), baked potatoes, white rice, processed cereals, and an endless variety of low- or no-fat desserts and candies—we now find at the top of the glycemic index. In sanctioned ignorance we ate our way to being overweight.

For people who recognize that losing weight and keeping

it off is a matter of life or death, diets that severely restrict fat succeed because the dieter is totally dedicated. Dieters feel wonderful, find a resurgence of energy, and a joy in life.

For most Americans, these diets are simply too extreme to work well.

DIETS THAT ARE CHIEFLY CONCERNED WITH INSULIN PRODUCTION

These diets are generally soundly based on the glycemic index of foods and the fattening chain reaction that occurs when high levels of sugar reach the bloodstream quickly. They rightly distinguish between complex carbohydrates and simple carbohydrates and urge an increase of the former and decrease of the latter.

They attempt to sort out what went wrong when we tried—and even succeeded—in cutting fat consumption in general and saturated fat consumption in particular.

They are probably more successful with more people than the rigidly reduced fat-content diets. Many of them are easy to use and easy to stay on because they pay more attention to eating well than eating less. Almost all are slight variations of a 30-20-50 plan (percentage of calories from: fat, protein, carbohydrates).

Among proponents are famous names like Nathan Pritikin, Adelle Davis, Richard Podell, Oprah Winfrey, and other authors of a series that have been bestsellers.

Not all of these limit calories, but some do. For a serious athlete, often those limits are insufficient. For instance, 30% protein in a 2000 calorie diet (as Barry Sears proposes in his Zone books) equals 600 calories from protein or 68 kilograms. If an athlete consumes that amount of protein in a 2000 calorie diet he or she is not getting enough carbohydrates. In addition, the high consumption of protein drains away body stores of water. It drops weight fast, but for the wrong reasons.

DIETS THAT STRESS FOOD COMBINING AND OTHER SINGULAR PRACTICES

No single food—grapefruit, cabbage, broth, or juice—has a secret fat-burning ingredient. The closest thing on earth to a fat-burning machine is sustained exercise.

There is no scientific evidence to support William H. Hay's 1930s notion that isolating one food source from the other produces weight loss or weight stabilization. This food combining simply starves your body alternately of simple carbohydrates, complex carbohydrates, protein, and fat.

Hay's idea found favor in the six-week Beverly Hills diet in the early 1980s and still finds followers. Since then we've had Hollywood diets of grapefruit; hospital-based, presurgical diets of cabbage soup, and a spate of similar wonder-food diets. Most often these lay out a day-to-day menu of designated foods and amounts. Many start fairly close to starvation levels and build to more normal meals that a dieter can live with long-term.

It's all smoke and mirrors. Most plans so severely reduce calories in an initial phase that dieters lose from six to 12 pounds in initial weeks. But much of this is water loss from restricting carbohydrates. It comes back quickly with normal carbohydrate consumption.

All probably work if followed religiously, but none does much to show the dieter how to eat normally and maintain the loss. Nevertheless they are quick; they take no thought or calorie counting; they propose ordinary healthy foods (just, sometimes too little of them); they are not expensive.

Conversely, they probably don't supply needed nutrients during initial diet periods; dieters are probably often hungry and bored; they eventually fall off.

Any diet that relies heavily on pills to the omission of natural foods or exercise is potentially either dangerous or a sham.

OTHER WEIGHT REDUCING TECHNIQUES

Surgical techniques such as stomach stapling, shortening the bowel, tummy tucking, and peeling away subcutaneous fat, can reduce severe problems, but they are not without complications. People get fat from eating too much, eating the wrong foods, and being sedentary. Pills and surgeries don't change habits and without changing habits few Americans can stay trim.

SO, WHAT ABOUT ME?

It's true that some people seem to be slim and to stay slim easily and some seem to gain pounds looking at a piece of chocolate cake. New research is recognizing such differences. One line of inquiry is tying life-time weight to in-utero nutrition and birth weight, but it still hasn't figured out what's good and what's bad. In addition, not one of us can do anything about how much or how well fed or undernourished we were as fetuses. Nor can we change how we were fed as children.

Although these factors may be important to study and may yield invaluable guidelines for future generations, they don't help us control our weight now. So we have to play with the cards we've been dealt.

In 90% of the cases of people who claim to gain weight on few calories, keeping an honest and complete food log is enlightening. By amounts, timing, and choices, people may be consuming calories that are likely to turn to fat. As simple a procedural change as eating a large meal at noon and lightly a few hours before bedtime can make a difference.

Almost all nutritionally based diets advocate three meals a day and two light snacks. Everyone agrees that spreading food intake out more evenly is advantageous. It's an additional technique to control blood sugar level and feel satisfied. The danger of this technique is that meals can stay the same and snacks can get out of hand. Monitor this carefully. In addition, heed to every diet advocate of the past century—don't skip breakfast.

Remember that you can and should establish a caloric-intake guide for yourself. Then, either very strictly or roughly, count calories for two weeks. You'll soon learn how to eat within your limits and, maybe more important, where you fall off the wagon.

That is the current basis of Weight Watchers. Its strength is that it establishes values for foods and regulates portions. For many dieters applying those factors and the social aspect of Weight Watchers is perfect. Its weakness is that although it acknowledges the importance of exercise and encourages it, its program is not as strong in this aspect as it could be.

We have a walking friend who over four months lost 34 pounds on the Weight Watchers program. That may be a little too much too fast (two pounds a week is a healthy goal). Julie, however, is walking vigorously and long, so her level of exercise may allow that increased loss. She says, "I like the program because it doesn't tell me I can never have another bag of potato chips or milk shake. It simply reminds me that if I have those, I have to cut back somewhere else.

"My husband is supportive—he doesn't mind the meals I'm now crafting. My daughter is very supportive; she thinks it is great that I can get back into tight bluejeans. My son thinks the whole thing is weird. I guess, however, that I'll just have to live with that, because I feel great."

Very generally, for a woman exercising moderately (walking or running 12-18 miles a week, playing tennis or swimming for three hours) taking in between 1800 and 2200 wisely chosen calories a day is healthy. For a man that range is between 2500 and 3000 calories.

But eating wisely is as important as eating moderately.

> Eating fruits, vegetables and whole grains is vital to good nutrition. Eating all plant foods as close to unprocessed as possible or raw is best.

> Limiting saturated fats is essential, but eating some omega-3 (walnuts, cold-water fish oils, flaxseed oil) and omega-6 (corn oil, canola oil, and so on) fats is as essential.

> Eating carbohydrates—mostly complex carbohydrates from plant sources—fat and protein on a 50-30-20 (carbohydrate, protein, fat) percentage basis or a 60-30-10 basis is important. Eating fiber is too.

> Drinking six glasses of liquids (mostly water) gives the body the medium it uses to circulate nutrients and regulate body temperature and waste.

(A word here about the glycemic index. This is a scale, developed over the past 20 years, that ranks foods by how quickly their carbohydrates raise the blood sugar. It was developed as a guide to diabetics and has been enlightening in many ways. In some it has yielded surprises, but, in general, it confirms that a rise in blood sugar is determined by:

> The kind of carbohydrate contained,

> The amount of fiber contained,

> The size of particle swallowed, and

> The amount of fat contained—which slows stomach emptying.

The scale is interesting, but it must be coordinated with serving size to be more generally useful. It is a great help, however, to any athlete or dieter and essential for any diabetic. It's forefront research and the best way to keep up with it is to use the Internet. A simple glycemic index search produces abundant and good information.

Finally, there only two scientifically proven, time-tested, healthy ways to lose pounds and keep them off:

> Restrict calories

> Exercise

Chapter 7

Setting Up A Routine

While spending for health clubs, home exercise equipment, and personal trainers is at an all-time high, more and more children and adults are overweight and unhealthy. Why?

The answers are simple; the solutions are complex.

Most Americans don't eat right and even many who spend money on fitness don't train right. They become bored, injured or quit for other reasons.

No diet will change American's love of fast food. Fast food, snacking and a sweet tooth cause most of our weight gain. To slim down, either we are going to have to live without fast foods (highly unlikely given the pace of our society) or fast foods will have to change because we demand it.

If we abandon McD and KFC and the likes for Subway, McD and KFC will get the message. But if double bacon cheeseburgers, fried chicken nuggets, and french fries continue to outsell grilled chicken, lean burgers, turkey sandwiches, and parsleyed new potatoes, we'll get the former.

McDonald's is great at public relations. Late in 2002, it grabbed headlines by announcing that it would eliminate transfatty oils in its french fries.

True, eliminating transfatty oils is good, but does it deserve headlines in every major newspaper in the country? Let's hope it educated some people about the danger of the oils they consume in many other ways (in margarine, baking mixes, prepared baked goods). However, the fast-food change prompts the question of why McDonald's was using transfatty oils in the first place. To understand let's look at these oils.

Transfatty oils are those which are hydrogenated. They are liquids that have extra hydrogen blown into them for two purposes: to turn a liquid into a solid or to extend the shelf-life of a product by retarding rancidity.

The former we use so that a liquid, such as corn oil, can come in a stick or in a plastic container that imitates butter. It also satisfies our Crisco-fetish in baking.

The latter we do so that crackers, some prepared cereals (granola), baking mixes and the like can stay on the grocery shelves or our shelves much longer without turning rancid.

Why, however, McDonald's—which needs a liquid oil to deep fry foods—was using a transfatty oil is not clear. Its french fries don't need shelf-life. It must have hydrogenated its oil to make it into a solid or semisolid state to increase its shelf life. Yet with millions of gallons used daily, the oil shouldn't need to sit around the McDonald's kitchen for weeks or months before use.

Thank heaven someone looked at that since it's now clear that transfatty oils are as bad for us as natural saturated fats. We should avoid them, but that's hard to do because of their use in so many products that need shelf life. We can, however, serve liquid olive oil with our bread (as many Italian restaurants are now doing) instead of using a tub or stick of margarine. There are also health-wise products that offer semisolid margarines without transfatty oil.

Eating right is not a matter of dieting, it is a long-term, everyday commitment to eating foods as natural as possible (whole grains rather than refined grains, raw fruits, raw or crispy steamed vegetables, leaner meats, all without heavy sauces, dips, or condiments) and avoiding fats.

We've already talked about Dean Ornish's diets, which drastically reduce fat. They are wonderful, proven, healthy diets that can help repair heart disease, as well as avoid it. There are none better tested and documented scientifically and proved successful. But they are too rigid to be followed long term by the average American—one whose life does *not* immediately depend on their benefits.

If you can live with under 20% fat in your diet, do so. However, research indicates that a diet that includes 30% fat is more sustainable for North Americans. Aim for that. You may be able, as an athlete, to reduce that percentage later.

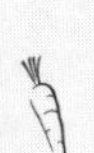

Remember, when it comes to food, less is almost always better—less refinement, less preparation, less fat, less sugar, fewer calories, less quantity.

When it comes to physical activity, more is always better—longer, farther, faster, harder, oftener. You do not have to be a competing athlete to be fit, but it always helps.

Training right means developing a weekly routine that combines training for strength, flexibility and aerobic conditioning. That routine must be varied—to avoid boredom and injury—but ironclad. It must be as vigorous as your goal demands or time permits. You must set priorities: conditioning your body must be close to the top, perhaps preceded only by family and work.

If you intend to become an athlete you need a smart training program. That program will work with your natural abilities. Each of us, even the most klutzy, has them. You may be a natural sprinter or distance competitor or someone whose quick reaction time and balance gives you an advantage in competitive sports.

Science has proved that the slow-twitch and the fast-twitch ratio of muscle differs from individual to individual. It has also verified that the pain threshold differs from individual to individual and, perhaps because of a physiological imperative—such as a high retention of muscular oxygen—that contributes to competitive success. Aerobic training in youth (working hard, playing hard at any sport) builds a lifelong base for healthful, physical activity. Being a computer addict, a bookworm, or a couch potato doesn't. That said, however, remember: *it is never too late to start.*

Not too many years ago, professional coaches believed that to be a better baseball player, you played baseball constantly. To be track star, you ran, exclusively. To be a better anything, you did more and more again of that activity. Only boxing coaches recognized that overall fitness made better boxers.

Today all professional athletes recognize the advantage of overall fitness. Exercise increases blood flow and muscle strength; these build endurance; endurance fights fatigue. Other things being equal, the athlete who is most alert longest wins the contest.

However, Ed warns that no one enjoys serious training. There are those braggadocio Ironman competitors who contend that they really don't train that long or that hard. No honest competitor, however, belittles his or her effort, understates the hours of training or claims to enjoy working as hard as he or she must work to get there.

At its inception, the Ironman competition in Hawaii signed up anyone who wanted to come. Before 1983, race directors were happy to have anyone who took up the challenge. But after the initial lark of racing those distances, participants learned that swimming 2.4 miles, biking 112, and running 26.2 was not for the untrained.

In 1979 the competition was discovered by the national media: *Sports Illustrated* gave this "lunatic" race its first major attention. In 1982 ABC's *Wide World of Sports* caught Julie Moss, *a professional athlete,* crawling across the finish line.

Totally depleted of energy, she "hit the wall" just before the finish line. She was, then, leading the women. As she came into the home stretch and stumbled into the lights and sounds of the finish line, the camera caught her. She staggered forward on legs that looked like rubber. She fell, she crawled forward. She waved off hands that would help her. She got to her feet, managing by sheer force of will to stumble a few steps forward before her legs again gave way.

As she fought her way forward, she was passed by Kathleen McCartney. Moss's struggle repeated itself again and again. She covered the last ten yards to finish 29 seconds behind McCartney.

Throughout the following day, from morning to last news, millions of viewers watched the spectacle of the Ironman. They gasped, held their breath, reached out emotionally, and finally breathed a long sigh as she fell over the finish line and collapsed into waiting arms.

The reality of the feat was established. No athlete thereafter undertook it lightly. Even today, however, in Hawaii there are a hundred DNF's (Did Not Finish). Most overestimated their ability and underestimated the grueling heat and distance.

In St. Louis, Deeds Fletcher, an early participant, yearly recruited friends, family and other slightly-wacky athletes to enter with him. They didn't have to qualify; when he started, the race was wide open and thereafter the race director took his word that those he brought would not embarrass him (or her). He went out of his way to represent the reality of the challenge and to help train those he recruited.

One friend tells this story of his first try. He had been training with Deeds for months. Deeds helped him join the small training circle and prepare for the race mentally. Our friend's wife and preteen children were well aware of the arduous program he undertook and stuck with religiously. He was absent from home for long hours. At least one day of the weekend they saw little of him. That was the day of the long, long workout on bike or foot and, eventually, bike *and* foot.

Although he was somewhat reticent to trumpet his intention widely, his children shared no such compunction. To attend, they would be absent from school for more than a week; they told everyone their dad was doing the Ironman in Hawaii. They never passed up an opportunity to explain exactly how great an athletic feat that was. Their pride runneth over.

When the family arrived in Hawaii, their father convened a family meeting. He warned them that he had never tried this before. He had prepared as best he could and thought that he was ready, but the day would be hot and the race would be, for him, very long. If he finished, he said, he would come in long after dark. And, he concluded, he might not finish.

"Not finish!" his children shrieked. What did he mean, he might not finish? They had told everyone he was doing the Ironman. How could they go home and say that their dad did not finish. How embarrassing! Surely he couldn't do that to them!

So he finished. And he went back twice, much to the satisfaction of his offspring, who always loved both Hawaii and their bragging rights before and after.

If serious training is never fun, why do it? Ed says there are some aftermath highs and on certain days you feel very good about being fast or strong or unbeatable. It's a feeling we seldom equal in everyday life. And the bragging rights are great.

But serious training is just plain hard work. While you are out there slogging away in the heat of the day, you aren't having fun. You do it not for race results so much as to increase the length and quality of your life.

And you do it too, to be a good example. You do it to teach your children, grandchildren, spouse, friends, colleagues that good health is everything in life.

For Ed, it's also part of his mission as a physician. He teaches and preaches that exercise is as important to mental as to physical health. It contributes not only to the participant's quality of life but to that of his or her whole family. He preaches that a dedication to exercise brings health, wealth and happiness.

All of that said, your choice of your physical activity will influence your enjoyment and success. If you are competitive, you'll need to win sometime. Hats off, then, to age-related competitive categories: masters competitions, seniors tours and Senior Olympics.

If competition isn't your thing, push yourself to the edge of your sport in endurance; swim for miles, bike toward a yearly goal or a long organized event, walk a marathon, have an overwhelming and perfect garden.

Dorothea walks marathons—slowly. Several times in St. Louis, she was the last marathoner to cross the finish line and in both cases she won first place—for runners and walkers—in her age group. Remember, it is never too late.

As the only woman in her age-group, her last would be first so long as she finished. Always think positively. Look at what ordinary Americans have accomplished in the past 25 years. In 1975, who among adults walked, jogged, ran, cycled, or swam on a regular basis? Only a few. Today millions do.

We have a 76-year-old friend who biked 4000 miles last year (she keeps a journal—always a must for competitive, compulsive athletes) and walked a marathon (albeit slowly, but to a trophy). Last year in the Senior Olympics, she entered power walking. On the first lap she was dead last. In the end she won a silver medal.

Her base-level fitness is so high that when the competitive spirit kicks in, she is able to shift into overdrive. She has the endurance to outlast less well trained athletes. When you are keeping fit, that accomplishment alone is fantastic. You are among the elite of any age. If you set a moderate standard and meet it, you are in the top 10% of your age group. Think of what that would have meant in academic performance and bring the same pride to physical performance!

Some time ago the *Wall Street Journal* noted that Bill Milliken, a 1960 Olympic gold medalist swimmer, swims almost daily. He is an exception. An estimated half of all former college and high school swimmers do not swim regularly.

Milliken offered these guidelines for any athlete:

> Measure your performance. Ignorance of how well or badly you do now is not bliss. It keeps you from competition and, eventually from working out altogether.

> Measure yourself only against others your age and sex.

> Never let a stranger intimidate you. In the swimming pool, in the weight room (where Milliken is a regular to avoid muscle and bone loss), anywhere, never feel inferior. You are exceptional by any standard.

> Turn strangers into friends to form a support group. You cheer their performance and they yours.

Remember the most important requirements for lifelong health are to stick with your regimen of physical activity and eat wisely. To do so you need to feel good about yourself and what you are accomplishing. And, you will, if you are faithful to yourself.

The latest surgeon general's report, as well as the latest guidelines from the American College of Sports Medicine, urge us to engage in a moderately taxing physical activity for 30 minutes a day, at least five days a week. Late in 2002, the government revised those figures to suggest a minimum of an hour a day.

More is always better. There is, however, a question of goals that are reasonable for you.

It's hard to imagine a mother or father of several small children, each parent with a full-time job, finding five hours a week to exercise. But it's not impossible.

Think then in terms of developing some family activities that are taxing:

> Put the little ones in backpacks and hike for a couple of hours. Carrying that extra weight is bound to be aerobic. If the kids are older, let them join in, it's also never too early to begin to strengthen muscle and heart.

> Do the same on bicycles. Bring a picnic.

> Use the weight room while the kids are at swimming lessons.

> Athletic fields often are parts of schools or community athletic complexes. Keep one parent on the sidelines cheering and free the other to do something aerobic.

> Turn everyone out for an session of basketball, volleyball, field hockey or soccer, swimming, sledding, skiing, skating, or just plain walking. Don't excuse Mom, or little sisters, or baby brothers. Have Dad pack the youngest on his back.

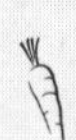

Every good routine has these three goals: resistance training, flexibility and aerobic fitness. Resistance training—some form of push against resistance—is usually isometric or isotonic. Flexibility is sustained stretching to keep muscles, tendons, and joints balanced and well used. Aerobic training is activity to the point of stress (breathing hard, increasing your heart rate, raising a light sweat, demanding more of your muscles).

This physical activity has to be an integral part of your everyday life. Develop a varied plan (what activities you will engage in, how often, how long, and to what intensity).

Vary your activity, but stick with it as if your life depended on it, because it does.

If you mean to compete, plan a routine week but also plan the pace and timing to bring you to a peak at the competition. Your weekly routine will maintain you at a high level of fitness, but not at the top. It will be your base for building both endurance and speed.

But remember that few of us can push ourselves to 24/7 training. A day of rest will help you rebound. Set a realistic goal to begin with, you can always do more; setting too high a standard is likely not only to have you do less, but to quit in frustration.

Slack periods are important. So is—if you'll recall from earlier chapters—Freud's "regression in service to the ego." (Your ego wants to be as comfortable as possible, to avoid stress and strain, to indulge in everything easy. When you repress that urge by self discipline—that is, when you do things like exercise that are good for you but hard—your ego suffers. Freud said that it is healthy to skip the hard things once in a while, just to satisfy your ego, to "service" it. If, every once in a while, you throw it a bone, you'll be better able to keep it leashed.)

You get increased performance only from stressing the muscle and bone and thereby building their capacity. It doesn't happen overnight. It takes weeks, months and years. If someone offers a six-week program, don't just beware, be disbelieving.

Unfortunately time is always working against you. The older you are the harder it is to build muscle strength and the easier it is to lose it by disuse. At 20, once you are in great shape for it, you can run 100 yards flat out every other week and maintain your capacity to excel, but at 40 that won't happen. To maintain a top level you'll have to run it flat out every week and work on it with less intensity every third day or so. At 60, if you want to go flat out on May 15, you will start building on your base on January 15.

In the serious competitor, only resistance training ensures balance. In developing a routine, you must pay attention to strengthening muscles that oppose the muscles you overdevelop by practicing your sport.

The most common long-term injury to runners involves the knee. There is a lesson in balance in this; it involves carefully strengthening the vastus medialis to keep the knee balanced in its socket.

The knee is kept in place by two large muscles: the vastus lateralis on the outside (which is really three muscles) and the vastus medialis on the inside (a single muscle). The repetitive activity of running strengthens the vastus lateralis. That strengthening pulls the knee out of its socket with the thigh bone.

Over time, in runners, this misalignment is responsible for 90% of all knee injuries. (The cartilage cushion of the knee is evenly distributed over the entire groove. If the knee is pulled outward by the stronger vastus lateralis, that cushion is worn unevenly and may eventually be worn away entirely.)

Every runner (or walker) must strengthen the vastus medialis to keep the knee aligned. This is done by two exercises; both can be done with or without aid of machine: Sitting on the edge of a surface, with a stiff leg, externally rotate the foot and raise the leg from the hip.

Then on a machine that weights the foot or using an improvised weight at the ankle (a plastic bag with a couple of cans of vegetables or a regular ankle weight) sit on the end of a surface with the knee bent. Raise the leg 90 degrees. Now lower to 60 degrees and bring back to 90 degrees repeatedly. (You can watch the inside muscle work during both these). The vastus medialis is engaged only in the last 30% of that 90 degree movement, so you don't have to lower all the way. Play between 60 degrees and 90 degrees.

Resistance training is as important to non-athletes. It gives older adults the skills to continue independent living. Even 90-year-olds improve greatly in muscle strength with six weeks of a solid daily program. So strength-training is a vital part of everyone's weekly physical regime. As a competitive athlete, you must do nearly as much of it as of competition-specific training.

The aerobic component of your training routine is the key to cutting risk of cardiovascular diseases. It is key also to endurance because your heart-lung capacity and the vascular network that supplies energy to the muscles determines your endurance. The blood supply—the ability of your body to deliver oxygen and carry away waste—determines when your body, or even a particular set of muscles, fatigues.

Only in long endurance events will you call on outside sources for nutrition. Although heat will mediate need, in general, in any event under two hours, your body will depend on stored energy. Aerobic conditioning builds that storage capacity.

Aerobic conditioning is also your tool for weight control. After the first 10 minutes of stressful activity, your body abandons carbohydrates as its main fuel and turns to stored fat. That means that for weight control, longer sessions are more helpful than shorter ones.

Flexibility and balance avoid the musculo-skeletal injuries that commonly follow aerobic and resistance training. Stretch before a race to loosen muscle and tendon and warm them up. Stretch after a race to relieve the tightness you have built by the repetitive, strained movement and also to improve circulation to carry away the lactic acid that caused muscle fatigue.

If you train wisely (and eat right), your body will give you competitive age-group times. Begin by setting goals. Do you want to run a marathon at 50; swim a mile; race walk; bike across Kansas; enter a kick-boxing competition; win in Senior Olympics; compete in a master's golf circuit; enter a triathlon? Anything goes.

Your ultimate goal is fitness, good health, more and better years, but you'll get there by setting your sights on short-term competition. If you are not competitive, set a doable goal to enter a taxing event and finish.

In most cases, however, you need more than one short-term goal. Often competition has a season, but if you are free to travel, that season may never end.

In the U.S. half-marathon or marathon run/walks and triathlons move north in the summer and south in the winter. If you want to widen your scope, pick competitions abroad (there are wine-country marathons in France every September, beer fests in Germany, Ironman Japan, the Honolulu marathon). What better way to see the world and put off forever having to join "seniors" tours.

Serious training needs to be year-round with different periods of intensity and duration. This is called periodization and will be discussed later at greater length. It changes your program at regular intervals. It gives flexibility because it changes many training variables in conjunction with your long-term goals. The period sets the goals appropriate for that stage of training.

Remember these basic training principles:

- *Overload.* The body must be stressed beyond its normal capacity to increase performance or muscle size and strength. In resistance training, weight resisted should be at least 60% of the maximum amount you can lift at one time.
- *Rest.* Gains can only take place when muscle groups are allowed sufficient time to recover between training sessions. In general allow 24 to 48 hours for any muscle group recovery.
- *Specificity.* To see adaptations that lead to improved ability at a specific task, you need to do that task and train for its specific requirements. You don't do sprints to run a marathon.

> *Variation.* To reach the maximum performance, you need to do a variety of exercise routines. You need to periodize for light, moderate, heavy days and weeks and, even, months. You need to vary activities.

> *Individualization.* To be best for you, your training needs to address your strengths and weaknesses. It needs to be structured to your goals, taking into account your prior history of injury or performance.

Chapter 8

Avoiding Injury

> **To avoid injury:**
>
> **> Cross-train;**
>
> **> Emphasize balance;**
>
> **> Stretch;**
>
> **> Take every preventive precaution.**

Those basics are under your control. Accidents happen; we are not always in control. It is a rare triathlete who has not had a serious bicycle accident, but being in shape enough to withstand the shock and recover is, to some extent, within your control. Pray that you won't encounter serious accident, but know that even in those circumstances, fitness can mitigate the injury.

In addition, follow the rules. Don't ride or blade without a helmet and padding; don't bat without a helmet; don't play hockey or soccer without headgear and eye and mouth protection. Other sports have other precautions. Observe them.

The very essence of the Ironman—cross-training—is its ultimate weapon against fatigue and injury. Seldom in the history of the race in Hawaii have accidents knocked a competitor out of the race. I know of no major swimming or running accidents, although rumors of shark presence in Kailua Bay are frequent.

(Somehow, however, the thrashing of 3000 strong arms in an Ironman mass start seems more likely to scare off a shark than attract one. Indeed, the possibility of a knock on the head or an elbow in the face in that seething mass of anxious humanity is far more likely. Of the approximately 1500 men and women who enter the water at 7 a.m. on those October mornings, all are accounted for in the long run.)

Just a word. In a mass start, you're bound to be beat up some. Having goggles knocked loose is the most likely, but swallowing a good deal of lake or ocean is also inevitable. Be understanding, but if someone persists in plaguing you, strike back. An elbow or a foot in the armpit or gut sends a message. Or you may want just to hang back a little. It's a long race.

In triathlons, bike accidents are frequent. Most of these are individual or two-bike derailments. The crosswind is always fierce on the King Kamehameha highway up the west coast from Kailua/Kona to the turn east to the long, long hill to Havi. In 1998, a dozen bikers arrived at the bike finish at the Kona Surf with bloodied right arms and legs. They had been blown over into the lava field enroute to Havi. All picked themselves and their bikes up, brushed off the cinders and went on full tilt. Volunteers in the changing tents at the Surf always have a supply of clean clothes and bandages. Showers are routine; by then—noon to early evening—the heat on that 112-mile black road is intense.

We have known competitors who came all the way to Hawaii only to be knocked out before race day by a severed heel or foot tendon. These were cuts from barnacles and sharp lava rock that make up much of the Big Island coastline. Good sturdy swim footgear is a safety must—for racers and families. (There are wonderful sandy public swimming and snorkeling beaches all along that coast, but venturing into other waters can be hazardous to the feet, as well as knees and elbows for the waves often slam an emerging swimmer into the rock.)

The Hawaii championship proves that because of the

intense cross-training, these are truly *iron* men and women. Such training increases strength and aerobic capacity faster than single repetitive activity. It allows for the intensity needed to do the Ironman.

Varying workouts also is a surefire strategy for weight control. When you work more muscles, you can exercise harder. As you vary activity, each set of muscles becomes more fatigue-resistant. At the same time, that variety is kinder to your body than when you push one activity hard.

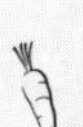

Most muscles adapt to repeated use in from two to four weeks. They become stronger almost immediately; but to build a better blood supply takes longer. As your muscles become stronger and blood supply increases your capacity takes a giant leap upward. Doing more, promotes doing more and variety is the key to staying injury free at this intensity.

It gives you rest with pluses. While you are recovering from high-intensity routines, you are benefiting in other ways—stretching and balancing in yoga or dance. Rest is not, then, a dead period.

Here's a basic *balanced* routine that takes an hour a day, six times a week. It's not sufficient for the serious athlete, but, gives a base to build on for competition:

Monday, run, walk, blade an hour—push it, include hills, or simulate that on a treadmill. This is a cardiovascular builder to increase strength and vascular delivery. According to Gabe Mirkin, M.D., dean of the sport physiologists, a 1% increase in grade, requires a 4% increase in energy. Your incline can be gradual, but long.

Tuesday, lift weights with a mostly upper-body routine. This is a day for strength training. Emphasize arm and back muscles, but also do some abdominal strengthening.

Use machines at home, but better, go to a club for social reinforcement. Spend 45 minutes to an hour, but vary activity.

Wednesday, do aerobic lower-body work: bicycle, spin, blade a hilly course, cross-country ski (inside or out) to raise your heart rate. If you swim, do so long and fast (swimming is almost lower-body neutral). Work at your own rate, but work a little harder each week.

Thursday, lay low with yoga, tai chi, some stretch and balance for a gentle hour. You need to stretch out the muscles you have been working and tightening. For best results reinforce this by taking a class.

Friday do a long, slow workout that combines upper body—swimming, rowing, kayaking, weights—and lower—running, biking, walking, blading. Don't push it; split it up if it suits you better. Play tennis, volleyball or basketball in early morning but do another low-impact, long, slow hour in the evening.

Saturday, weather permitting, get outside. Push yourself for strengthening and aerobic conditioning. Take advantage of your leisure for more than an hour. If you have family or friends who will join you make this a social affair. Go hiking and picnicking. If you are walking, use walking poles; they can add an upper body workout to burn as many as 25% more calories.

Sunday, do a low impact activity—ballet, Pilates-based class, or one of the gentle Asian arts—or just plain rest. If you are seriously training, however, you'll need this leisure day for your long, long workout. If that's what you intend, rest on Friday and come back strong for the weekend. Remember, you do need to rest. It gives muscles time to refuel with glycogen and get rid of waste.

Age will vary this routine somewhat. The older you are, the more rest you need. But that's the beauty of cross-training; you rest while you work. Swimming doesn't cause much lower-body strain, and if you wish to rest the lower body completely, disable it with a pull buoy that keeps your feet elevated. Weight work isn't much cardiovascular strain. Kayaking is all upper body and surfing is both. Like baseball or softball, golf is some upper body, some lower (if you walk and push a cart), but isn't enough strain to be considered cardiovascular. Do these just for fun and variety.

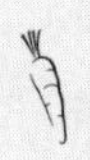

Remember: measure your performance. Always keep a journal. Avoiding that is a cop-out. That's why training partners and training groups are so important. But your goal is to be among the best athletes of your age, not to win the gold.

WEAK LINKS

Physical therapists swear that most sports injuries can be avoided by:

> Heeding warning signs, and

> Working to strengthen weak links.

Therapists are not, generally, talking about sudden injury from a fall or a collision but those injuries that develop over time from over- or mis-use: shinsplints that lead to stress fractures: achilles tendinitis in runners whose foot rolls in or out on impact; iliotibial band injuries from repetitive bending and straightening the knee or from uneven shoe wear; wrist tendinitis caused by overuse; tennis elbow cause by overuse and imbalance; back pain caused by imbalance and ab weakness; and, of course, the ever-disabling knee injuries.

All of these begin with warning signs. Ignoring them is ignoring your body's red light—pain. Sometimes weak links are anatomical. If your legs differ slightly in length; get orthotic shoe inserts to avoid lower-back or hip injuries. Sometimes weak links are caused by bad equipment or form. A tennis racket with too large a grip can lead to tennis elbow. Unevenly worn shoes can strain the iliotibial band. Sometimes your very activity is causing the problem. As we said earlier: You are always strengthening certain muscles and those strong muscles cause an imbalance if the corresponding (antagonistic) muscles are not strengthened. Remember the lesson of the exercises that stabilize the knee from pulling outward because running has strengthened the outer-knee muscles.

In a conditioned athlete, pain is not normal. You surely will feel soreness as you push harder, faster, longer, but persistent pain is not a normal part of exercising. If you feel pain, think about what you did. You may be uncovering a new weak link. If you have a new ache doing the same old thing, consider it the red light on your body's dashboard.

When you recognize a warning sign, back off. See if rest will cure it. If the pain gets worse or even just continues while you are resting, seek help.

The simplest line of help comes from fellow athletes. Chances are you are not inventing the problem. Others have experienced it and worked through it. Talk to others, see what they recommend. If you can't find an answer there, try the Internet.

The second line of help can be the professional at your workout place. See what he/she/they know. Once again, you are unlikely to be experiencing something unique. If you have a trainer, never fail to inform him/her of persistent or acute pain. Perhaps your routine is exacerbating the problem and needs changing.

Finally, see a sports-medicine doctor or sports physiologist not only to diagnose and treat the problem, but to recommend measures to head off repetition. Good physiologists—whether they are physicians, physical therapists, or trainers—are worth their weight in gold.

That's why Tim Meyer, a Ph.D. candidate in exercise physiology, is an advisor to this book. Health Professionals such as Tim are also invaluable in honing technique for a particular sport and setting up a balanced, workable exercise regimen.

IN GENERAL TO AVOID INJURY:

> Increase your training gradually. Up the intensity, frequency, and duration week by week, maybe even month by month (depending on your age), not day by day. Never do more than 10% of the last period.

> Listen to your body. Don't power through pain. Find out what's going on and do something about it before it disables you.

> Always work on stretch, flexibility, and balance. If you are right handed and probably right bodied, do more repetitions to the left than the right. Little things, like switching the sides you routinely lift or carry with, breathing on both sides while swimming, changing the foot you routinely lead with can make a difference.

> Consult an expert about any known weakness. Let him or her work out a preventive schedule before you push hard.

> Diagnose your trouble zones—weak abs; inflexible spine and back; hip, knee, and ankle flexation limitations; immobile iliotibial band; overpronation in running—as you go and immediately work to correct them. Remember, 90% of all lower back problems are caused by the inability of the abdominal muscles to stabilize the spine. Leg lifts and leg rolls are never easy, but always effective.

> Build strong abs. They fix (stabilize) the pelvis. That in turn permits the legs to be flexed on the pelvis. If the pelvis rocks with leg movement, legs flail and the gait becomes uneven. By destabilizing the entire rhythm of the gait, whole sets of coordinated muscle movements are thrown into chaos and fatigue easily.

> Particularly for endurance events, work on strengthening common weak links. In the Ironman run, a standard weak link manifests itself: neck muscle weakness. A wobbly head is a sure sign that a competitor isn't likely to finish. For any triathlete, strengthening the neck is a must. Staying in an aerodynamic tuck position on the bike, while keeping the head up, puts immense strain on the neck muscles. Imagine how that works out after 112 miles!

DIAGNOSING WEAK LINKS

You can use some yoga postures to identify weakness in your flexibility that can contribute to injury.

> Do a half-twist. Sit on floor, one leg out, the other bent, crossed over at the knee, foot flat. Turn away from the outstretched leg (turn right if your left leg is outstretched and vice versa). You should come close to turning at a right angle. Do both sides. If you cannot, work on spinal rotation with this posture and other twisting stretches.

> Try a deep squat, hands on hips. You should lower hips to knees with knees over feet without rounding the back. Otherwise try to increase flexibility of ankle, hip and calf.

> Try leg raises. Lie on your back, raise one leg 90 degrees, keep the other flat on floor. Do both. If you can't, strengthen back and abs with crunches and leg raises. Also do hamstring stretches.

> Do an inline lunge. Align legs one behind the other. With hands behind neck, lower the back knee to floor without

leaning forward or twisting. You need this flexibility and balance to handle quick weight shifts and changes of direction. It is terribly important if you are playing tennis, basketball, soccer, hockey, or rugby. Work on thigh flexibility and strength and balance.

A professional trainer or physiologist can help diagnose weak links. It's worth the effort because to compensate beforehand avoids injury.

Chapter 9

Stretching and Flexibility

We have a friend who at 45 was a world-class short-distance racer. He had the long, skinny body and loose limbs of a premium runner. His stride was so easy, you would swear it cost him no effort. In local and regional competition he was a legend.

Although his success seemed God-given, we knew that wasn't all of it. We would see him early in the morning in the park several days a week working on intervals. Once he retired, he trained every day. But, somehow more effort didn't give him better results. He was often injured. Friends tried to talk him into running longer at slower paces. He never mastered the long, slow workout.

However, no matter what his goal, he spent hours training. Even while he worked, he never failed to find the time. Yet finding 15 minutes to stretch was beyond his ken.

He was used to being very good; in stretching he was very bad. He could touch his toes if he bounced down quickly, but he couldn't sit down, stretch out, and reach and hold his toes, even one leg at a time. All of the muscles that propelled him forward at such speed kept him from the stretch.

He tried yoga and gave it up. He said he didn't have time. He said, moreover, that he couldn't do most of the asnas. It was true, he couldn't, which was the very reason that he should. Now, at 60, he doesn't run.

Stretching may be overlooked because it doesn't yield obvious, immediate benefits. Its results are long-term and negative—you avoid injury. Who gives you credit for being the most limber miler or tennis player in your group?

> **Stretching is perhaps the most under-used tool in the athlete's duffle. That makes so little sense as to be ridiculous. It is so important to lifelong performance that sustained stretching, such as yoga, must be a part of every training routine.**

Stretching also may be undervalued because for dedicated athletes, to begin with, it is hard. Stretching should be uncomfortable—you have to push a little to achieve a gain—but never really painful. However, that said, if you are really muscle bound and rigid, it may be somewhat painful initially. In the long run, however, if stretching is painful, it's probably being done incorrectly.

Never, never, push to the point of pain, only tension. When you begin, pain may be an aftermath, not a performance sensation. If a stretch is painful, back off a bit. Where you are is exactly where you should be. Work from there.

There's no right or wrong end result in yoga poses, only an ideal. Visualize the ideal and you'll come closer to it eventually. To be honest, however, some poses that seem simple may never come.

Stretching your hamstrings after years and years of building them to keep you erect is not easy. They are tough, so be grateful for small improvements. In women who have worn high heels since adolescence, the Achilles tendon may be so tight, they can't bend knees with heels on the ground. Be patient. Most stretches will come.

However, lifelong, you may be the worst student at a full forward bend and the best at a lotus position with upturned soles on thighs. Like everything else about you, stretching is individual.

Over time, stretching will reduce the risk of injury, lessen exercise-induced muscle soreness and improve performance. It is a long-term exercise. You will become more flexible over months, even years.

Alas, in age, although you have been faithful to your stretching, you will go the other way. Despite minor setbacks, staying as limber as you can, will have enormous rewards. You'll be moving like someone years younger than you actually are and loving it.

Human muscle is fascinating because it has built-in protective mechanisms to prevent tearing. Tiny stretch receptors within the working muscle fibers sense the degree of stretch. They relay this message across the spinal cord to the nerves that control the contraction. These receptors fire more rapidly and strongly as the intensity of the stretch increases. If that stretch exceeds a certain threshold, the stretched muscle will protect itself by contracting. This is the "stretch reflex."

In the body's usual fail-safe reaction, there is also an inverse stretch reflex. It involves receptors in the tendons. These are sensitive to the tension in the tendon (not the muscle). Activated by muscle contractions, these receptors also send messages via the spinal cord to the nerves controlling the contraction. But when they are activated, they actually inhibit the contraction to protect the tendon from tearing.

Stretching should always be gradual. If you overstretch or hold a hard stretch for too long, you activate the inverse stretch reflex. You can feel it: after about 60 to 90 seconds, the muscle "gives" to relax the tension.

There are four common stretching techniques: ballistic, passive, contract-relax, and static.

You may have done ballistic stretches in your high school gym class or team workouts. Remember when you bobbed up and down very quickly in warmups? These are done quickly, causing the stretch reflex to activate and the muscle to contract rapidly. They are counterproductive. Don't do the same thing now or ever. If your aerobics routine includes them, cut them out.

Passive stretching is beneficial for experts at stretching, but can be harmful for the inexperienced. In this, a partner applies external pressure to increase the extent of a stretch. It's done widely in gymnastics to achieve that incredible flexibility. Done right, it's extremely effective. Done to a beginner, it's dangerous.

In contract-relax stretching the muscle to be stretched is actively contracted first. In theory that activates the inverse stretch reflex, reducing the muscle tension during the subsequent contraction. In theory in this stretching, you contract, feel the "give-up" induced by the inverse stretch reflex, and then immediately stretch. But this doesn't work. Rather than reduce the subsequent tension of the stretch, it increases it. In a variant of the contract-relax technique, you contract the muscle antagonistic to the muscle that has just relaxed. It's an improvement, but not worth the effort.

Static stretching is the common stretch technique. The stretch is slow and gradual and held for from 30 to 60 seconds. Tension builds slowly and the stretch reflex is not activated. As the tendons are stretched gradually, the inverse stretch reflex is activated and muscle is then stretched a little farther as the tension falls. This seems the most effective form of stretching.

In a slow, static stretch, if the stretch is held overall for the same duration (say 60 seconds), holding the ultimate stretch for 10 seconds is as beneficial as holding it for 30 seconds. To get the most bang for your buck, build your stretch gradually, hold it at your maximum for 10 seconds, then back off a little and continue to hold that just-under-hurting stretch for another 30 seconds or more.

If you are starting from scratch, begin with short periods several times a week. Once you've reached the level of flexibility you feel is beneficial to your performance, you can drop back to a single weekly, hour-long practice. However, more will probably yield further flexibility.

For adequate benefit, set aside an hour a week for yoga stretches. But also stretch routinely, every day. It's easy. Make it a habit.

For workaday stretching, put aside the car phone, stretch your back at every stoplight, hold until it changes. Get a head-set and as you teleconference, put your hands up to the back of your neck, pull your elbows back, hold. Grab your wrists or elbows behind your back, pull your shoulders back, hold. With palms on the desk, push back, hold. Sitting at a table or desk, stretch out a leg, heel down, hold. Repeat with the other leg. Do the same toe down. As you stand in a line, do the leg stretches. As you sit anywhere in private, drop one arm toward the floor, raise the other over your head, with back straight, arch toward the floor side. In the car as a passenger do neck exercises. As the driver, do them at stoplights.

You don't have to be obvious about stretching; it's possible to be unobtrusive as you sit or stand almost anywhere. But if you have the luxury to be obvious, do so.

While standing in a line that is stalled, bend over, grab your ankles/toes, hold. If you've been sitting for a long time, use a window sill to bend from the hip and stretch out your entire back, heel to head, hold. When you get out of a car after a long ride, grab your elbows behind your back and lean backwards to reverse that hunched-shoulder slump. Always hold for at least a count of 10.

When you can, sit on the floor rather than in a chair or on a couch. The floor opens endless possibilities for stretching. If you spend 60 minutes watching world and local news, a game or video, sit on the floor and stretch. Hold the stretch for 30 to 60 seconds (14 to 18 breaths). Lean forward, touch your toes, head up to see. Put one leg out to the side, arch the opposite arm over your head, bend into the outstretched leg. Get on your knees, hands on buttocks, lean backwards. Put one arm up behind your head, elbow up, bring the opposite behind your back, try to touch (if you can't, use a strap, a sock, a towel, to pull hands together). Sit with legs out in front, push heels forward, tighten abs, stretch upward. With legs forward, bend knees, soles together, lean forward with a straight back. Sit on one leg, stretch the other out, lean back on your elbows. Invent other variations on routine stretches.

Every serious athlete's duffle should contain a sturdy strap—cloth or heavy rubber—for stretching. Any of the above stretches can be done with a strap. If you can't reach a handy body part—toes, wrists, knees, elbows—use a strap rather than bending and straining. If you can't reach your feet with a forward bend, anchor the strap on the bottom of your feet and pull forward keeping back straight. If on your stomach, you can't reach your ankles for a boat stretch, use the strap to pull your feet forward. Do the arm-behind-the-head, arm-behind-the-back stretch with a strap if you can't interlace fingers.

Other yoga stretch aids can be helpful. If you cannot reach the floor on side stretches or forward stretches, a sturdy block of styrofoam or wood can help. These give you an anchor rather than let you hang out there unsteadily. Putting your feet on a wall or resting legs on a chair behind you can help you do a reverse posture (feet overhead) you might not be comfortable in for starters otherwise. A headstand is the one posture that we believe is best done initially with an apparatus. (This is a four-leg stool that allows you to put weight on shoulders rather than head. It's expensive if you're contemplating home use, but can be homemade (use a picture of the real thing) for pittance with a little ingenuity—piping, wood blocks to hold the legs steady, and foam rubber for padding.)

If you want to try a headstand without an apparatus, put hands on the floor in front of you, knuckles to the wall. Put head on hands, elbows close in. Rise from knees to flat feet. Walk feet in until your lower back in on the wall. Raise legs one at a time or have someone help you get up (and, in the beginning, down). Balance against the wall. You'll eventually find your balance for a free-standing posture.

If you are not doing yoga with a class, buy a good, complete yoga book or tape(s) to learn the basic asnas (poses) and improvise to suit your needs from there. But also stretch in everyday activities.

For a successful flexibility program:

> Follow the program year round. Expect results after weeks or months.

> Stretch specifically before and after exercise. The increased flexibility that results from before-stretches can last for up to three hours.

> Start with easy stretches; build to more advanced stretches.

> Alternate to balance the muscles stretched.

> Don't continue a stretch that causes pain. Assume the stretch slowly and stretch to a slight tightness of the muscle. To achieve the maximum benefit, hold for 10 seconds, back off slightly, hold for 30 more.

We think joining a yoga class is a key to dedicating adequate time to stretching routinely and to sticking with it. Go with a partner if you can. It will keep you more honest in attendance.

Individualize your stretches according to your workout or sport. You'll find guides to sport-specific stretches in the magazines devoted to your sport or in training books. Runners' stretches aren't necessarily the whole routine for a tennis player. A runner needs to keep thigh muscles loose because he/she is tightening them constantly in a stride. That's not as important for a golfer. He/she needs to work more with upper back and arm muscles.

That said, however, every increase in flexibility helps your body cope with the overuse of training. Balance is king; work for it in stretching.

Chapter 10

For the Serious Competitor

Within a pyramid representing training, the base is aerobic; for a competitive athlete it would occupy the bottom third. The next third would be strength training (weights). The top would be sports-specific speed work. For a beginning competitor, however, there would be no top. You can't go anywhere without those bases.

Every competitive athlete lifts weights and does Nautilus training. That training not only builds sport-specific muscles, it increases endurance and heart capacity, prevents injuries by strengthening bone, as well as muscle, and—by increasing muscle perfusion—builds the oxygen-carrying capacity of the blood (dopes it).

If you are new to athletic competition, in the first six months, do a few races to satisfy yourself and see where you stand, but otherwise, stop. Don't do specific speed training. Even a seasoned athlete following periodization has a precompetition phase: a base that renews aerobic fitness and solidifies strength gains. Once past that, train for speed. Only in the last few weeks before a major event will you *abandon* aerobic workouts and strength training for speed work.

No matter what your competitive sport, for most of your training, one speed session a week will suffice. Kick that up about four to six weeks before your event. (When you begin serious speed training depends on the length of your competition and your age. Those will determine your taper.) On every—really *every*—workout, warm up and down. Quit while you still have some energy in the tank. Then cool down.

For running, biking, competitive walking and blading, hill training is essential. For other sports that depend on lower body strength, speed, and agility (tennis, soccer, basketball, baseball and the like) hitting the hilly road like a boxer isn't a bad idea either. It builds strength and endurance without subjecting you to pounding on the flats.

If you are competing in track, a track is the place for your work—but don't eliminate hill workouts. If you are heading for longer competitions, the track has only one advantage—it's measured. Otherwise, it is too hard a surface and boring, boring, boring. Head for grassy paths and woodsy settings.

FOR SPEED INTERVALS

On a short, gradual hill, run three, then six repetitions of 100 meters, 300, and finally 600. Lean slightly into the hill, but keep a plumb line perpendicular to the hill or you lose power, speed, and efficiency. On a steeper hill, cut those lengths to 75, 225, and 450 meters, but keep the repetitions. Always jog or walk back to the starting point.

Hill running is the best way to build running specific muscles. If you are training for an endurance run (even a half-marathon) hill training in your speed phase isn't necessary. The best way to build speed is tempo runs.

To do that, run at your lactate threshold (85 to 90% of your maximum heart rate). The longer you go in training (start with 20 minutes and for a month try to build to a maximum) at this threshold, the faster your race pace will be.

You are training specifically to diminish your body's production of lactate and to build its ability to process lactate. How fast you can do this and postpone the inevitable build-up that causes muscle fatigue depends on your blood supply. Your veins carry waste away. Lactic acid is a byproduct of the biological process that converts the oxygen in blood to energy.

Elite performers can sustain work levels substantially

above their lactate threshold for up to one hour. They do so because they have trained very hard specifically for their exercise task (biking, running, skiing). By doing this they have achieved a balance of production and clearance. Lactate production can be decreased by training, but it's also a high clearance rate you are after in pushing your lactate threshold in training.

When you begin training, your threshold is probably at about 60% of your VO2 max (maximal oxygen consumption). Usual training brings that up to 70%. Elite endurance athletes and top masters athletes generally have lactate thresholds at 80-90%; 90% is rare.

Between aerobic fitness and intense speed workouts is a cruise interval. A cruise interval can be used in running, biking, swimming, walking, sculling, cross-country skiing, and other individual sports. It involves doing longer intervals, with slightly lower intensity, but with the intense interval rest period. Its purpose is to build longer endurance at an exertion level just below the anaerobic threshold. It builds endurance and aerobic fitness but it also pushes speed.

On the bike, for instance, you would do a 15-minute push that raised your heart rate to high in zone 2 or low in zone 3 (see page 113). In cruise, you maintain the same rest as in intense (or tempo) intervals. The intense interval works strictly on speed; the cruise interval contributes less to speed and more to endurance. Do the cruise interval at lease once a week (aim for 10% of your weekly mileage) during routine training. Use the intense interval as the last step toward racing.

Fartlek training has been used by distance runners for years, but is equally applicable to other sports, even team sports. The word comes from the Swedish for speed play. It has evolved under different given names: Watson, Saltin, Astrand, Gerschler, and the generic Hill, Whistle and Games. In every case it is an intense interval, although each sport has a specific goal: for instance, the Watson Fartlek is designed for runs of 10k and under and cross-country, whereas the Gerschler Fartlek aims to increase fitness in a program of steady running, the Games Fartlek uses a variety of speed workouts including running, jogging, changing directions for soccer, field hockey, baseball, basketball, other team sports. It's generally designed sport-specific by a coach.

MONITORING TRAINING

No one trains smart without monitoring. If you have trained for anything, you know that how hard you work and how you feel don't always match. One day you breeze through a mile in six minutes; the next you struggle through in nine. Did you get good training in both?

You think that if the mile in six was so easy, you weren't building an aerobic base. But you also think that there was something wrong on that mile in nine. You think that probably wasn't good aerobic training either, although your heart was pounding and your shoulders were heaving most of the way.

Formally, this monitoring is called perceived effort. However else you monitor, never abandon this basic feedback. It is priceless, but responding inappropriately isn't training smart.

If you are training seriously and having a bad day, your got-to-get-these-miles-in reaction is probably to power through the session. That's wrong. Switch gears. Say to yourself, "Well my periodization says today is an aerobic building/stress session, but I think my body just said, 'not on your life.'"

Don't then turn on your heels and head for home. Say, "Well, here I am. Can I use this time wisely anyway?" Change your goal. Make this session a renewal session; lower the intensity, lay back, do your miles, enjoy being at harmony with your body. And think, think, think about what you've done in the past few days. How have you rested and how much? How have you eaten (and drunk)? How has work- and home-life gone so far as stress is concerned? How are your overall health and medication?

If you listen to your body, those awful, off days can teach you much. But in these days of technology, also don't ignore the opportunity to get more information.

> Use a heart-rate monitor. It doesn't have to be expensive, but learn to use all of the information it is giving you. It is monitoring physiological stress.

If you normally push yourself, it will keep you from overdoing. On the other hand, if you like to take it easy, it will probably challenge you to kick it up a notch.

> Establish your maximum heart rate (mhr). Don't assume anything. Go out hard and get a big number. Probably the best test would be a real one—race. Or use a treadmill: turn up the speed and the incline until you feel your lungs, heart and head will burst. Then stagger off and look. If you are just going to push it; try more than once and take the highest number.

If, however, you are afraid of that kind of stress, don't do any of that. Use an mhr formula instead. We recommend: 180 minus half your age. Then subtract 10 if you are a couch potato; subtract 5 for training of one to five years; add 5 for training more than five years.

Now, using that mhr establish five heart zones. Max zone (Zone 5) is 90 to 100%; anaerobic zone (Zone 4) is 80 to 90%; aerobic zone (Zone 3) is 70 to 80%; build zone (2) is 60 to 70%; and healthy zone (1) is 50 to 60%. Exercise at zone 1 is good for your heart; zone 2 begins aerobic conditioning; zone 3 steadily builds it; zone 4 crosses the anaerobic threshold; and zone 5 is as much strain as you want to put on your heart on a sustained basis.

Do your favorite workout. See at what level you are comfortable working. Whatever that is, push it up a zone to see if you can be comfortable there. Remember that as long as you are working at 50 to 60%, you are doing heart-healthy exercise. It simply won't do for competition.

FOR SERIOUS TRAINING

> Keep a training log. It will help jibe perceived effort with monitored effort. It will quickly show if you are pushing too hard and having a backlash or not pushing hard enough to reach a goal.

> Weigh yourself every day. Your training has two components for success: exercise and weight. If you work for months toward a competition, but go into it with more weight than you want, you are defeating yourself. A reliable scale tells you how your two tools are working together.

> Measure body fat. Body-fat calipers are inexpensive and relatively accurate. So are the new combination scale-body-fat analyzers (but most are not calibrated to give real accuracy to the serious athlete). Better than either is to have body fat tested occasionally at your workout place.

TAPERING

Since competitive athletes are compulsive people—and more specifically compulsive trainers—doing less or nothing may be, ironically, the hardest aspect of training to grasp as essential. Listen up! Tapering is *essential.*

Research has documented its benefits and answered many specific questions about what, when, how, and how much. It hasn't been very age specific. It has, however, confirmed that the older you get, the longer your recovery time, so adjust your taper to your age and the race distance.

For a major event, begin to taper two weeks before. In that first week reduce training to 66% and in the second take it down to 33%. A major benefit of tapering is healing and that may be healing injuries that you are not even aware of. When you train hard you punish your body. You stress it to become stronger and more efficient, but that hurts you too. So before a race, give yourself time to heal.

If you are heading for anything as stressful as an Ironman distance (generally 9 to 16 hours), begin to taper your running at least four weeks earlier. Begin a bike/swim taper about 10 days later. For this kind of event—whether it's ultra marathons or ultra anything else—you have been preparing for at least eight months. Be assured that pushing harder in the month before the event isn't going to build strength or endurance. So taper—cut your endurance/ strength training by 20% in week one, 40% in week two, 60% in week three, and 80% in race week.

That is not going to ruin you, because you will retain intensity. Intensity is the key to maintaining your status. When you begin to taper, don't reduce your interval training. As you get close to race day, keep up the interval hours but reduce the "on" time and lengthen the "off" time—push shorter, rest longer.

Know that it takes your body seven to 10 days to reap the benefits of physiological stress. Anything that you do in the last week isn't putting any cash in the energy bank. It's just withdrawing.

Well structured tapering allows you body to heal, blows off psychological stress, builds muscle glycogen stores, solidifies neuromuscular coordination at race pace, helps mental focus and actually "dopes" naturally by increasing blood volume—more blood carries more oxygen.

Why then do anything in the last week? Do a few short-duration, race-pace intervals so that you don't go completely crazy. You also want to stay loose, so a few short intense sessions can serve both purposes and keep your neuromuscular system comfortable with race pace.

In preparation for competition, you have also been glycogen-loading in your muscles—carbo starvation and then loading. If you push too much in the last few days, you are withdrawing those deposits. (See Chapter 11.)

Chapter 11

Fueling for Competition

Eating right is to race fueling what aerobic training is to race performance. Fueling for a competition no more begins a week, a month, or six months before than building an aerobic base. Fueling also means hydrating, so in the days before a race, drink lots of water (caffeinated coffee, tea, soft drinks —and alcohol—don't count).

First, despite their healthy habits, some athletes are notoriously poor eaters. If you use energy bars as a staple, forget it. Energy bars, gels and nutrient replacement drinks are training- and race-fare, not a balanced diet. (Perhaps the athlete who doesn't have a stable table—real meals—is an exception, but even then go lightly as possible.)

These supplements are not even essential, but may be helpful, as prerace fueling. On the morning of, say, an Ironman, when whole colonies of butterflies settle in, use them instead of an 800-calorie breakfast to reload glycogen in the liver.

Since a section of this book dealt with nutrition, there's little left unsaid about a healthy diet. But some of it bears repeating.

One hard and fast rule: protein does not translate across the board into muscles, no matter what the old-time trainers or new-time diet proponents claim. Don't load protein to build muscle.

Too often health-conscious athletes pick out a dozen healthy foods and eat them day in and day out. Yuck! Bagels, turkey breast, tuna, green salads, pastas, low-fat yogurt, skim milk, and bananas do not a healthy diet make—even supplemented by energy bars and vitamins and minerals. If these diets make life simple, they make eating boring and that's a crime. Being an athlete does not call for nutritional deprivation. Far from it. Variety is its key.

It does, probably, call for fast-food deprivation. In *Triathlete* magazine, Scott Tinley wrote about deciding to have a double-bacon cheeseburger—or the like. Come to think of it, he probably wouldn't have the bacon even if he indulged in the juice-oozing hamburger topped with cheese. At any rate, he couldn't remember when he had last had one and since he wasn't training hard, maybe he deserved to lapse. He spent a long time talking himself out of it, then ordered it and took it home. Thereafter he lost interest. I don't remember if he craved french fries too, but we would.

We came to the conclusion—as he evidently did—that he did deserve to lapse. Remember Freud's "regression in service to the ego." However, don't do it on the nights before a competition.

For the competitive athlete a 60% carbohydrate, 20% protein, and 20% fat diet is often recommended. Fool with these percentages a little to suit yourself. This is more carbohydrate and less fat than we recommend for the average American diet (closer to 50/20/30). It is surely more fat than the best heart-healthy diet (10% fat). It is, thank heaven, far less protein than in faddish high-protein diets.

Competitive athletes need carbohydrates; they are basic fuel of movement. And they need fat, to replace fat—which they burn in all long events—without adding overall body fat. The longer the race, the more fat you need; however, fat does not metabolize normally without carbohydrate, so you need both. That's what 60/20/20 does. Athletes need protein to build muscle and bone, but not nearly the level high-protein diets recommend.

In all of this, experiment. Try a minor race with more protein and less carbohydrate. No one else's body is exactly like yours. Just don't experiment in the two weeks before an important event.

This advice, however, has one caveat: as you taper, reduce calories—particularly fat.

If you have been going all out, you could eat like a hog. You haven't, of course. You have chosen carefully most of the time, but you've been able to consume enormous numbers of calories. When you cut back training, if you don't cut back calories, you'll pick up pounds. Be careful.

Remember two healthful diet essentials:

> Eat foods as naturally as possible. Eat whole, less-processed grains, raw or crispy steamed fruits and vegetables, salads without heavy dressing; drink plenty of water.

> Eat a variety of foods—20 or 30 different foods a week.

Natural foods retain most of the vitamins, minerals and enzymes. All processing loses some of these, particularly enzymes and water-soluble vitamins. Select the freshest foods possible; real farmer's markets and roadside stands are a boon. You will then do as well as you can without growing your own. If you have time and inclination, don't rule that out. Gardening is, after all, exercise.

"Natural" can also mean foods grown organically. Choosing these avoids a major problem of our factory-food industry—the presence of foreign substances in and on our foods.

Hats off to the quality of our supermarket produce. We haven't had such quality available since we left the farm, and we haven't had such variety ever before. (The farm housewife was hard pressed to serve 20 or 30 different foods during a long winter and did so only by home canning. It diminished the nutritional value, but enhanced other aspects of family nutrition.)

Vegetarianism isn't incompatible with athlete nutrition; it simply takes more planning and imagination. New soy products make this easier since the major challenge of vegetarianism is to get complete proteins.

Variety is not only the spice of life and diet; it's nature's medicine chest.

Variety widens our supply of nutrients. Kiwi has as much vitamin C as an orange, some unusual enzymes and plenty of potassium; apricots have beta carotene and vitamin C; bananas load potassium; grapes and raisins supply iron. If you ate only bananas, you'd miss the cancer-fighting antioxidant beta carotene. In addition, bananas have little fiber —which apples have in abundance—and a high glycemic index (the index of how fast a food raises your blood sugar).

Variety also prevents the buildup of any harmful agent. If your grapes have a high residue of a pesticide (which can carry over to their raisin form) and you only eat grapes and raisins, you'll be ingesting much of that pesticide.

Variety also reduces your need for supplements. However, we can't think of an athlete (or, for that matter, almost any other American) who doesn't take supplements. It's a rather-be-safe-than-sorry phenomenon. In addition, athletes, by their very athletics, build free radicals; antioxidants are the antidote.

Our foods contain 600 known compounds: vitamins, minerals, enzymes, fiber, fat, carbohydrate, protein, phytochemical and probably trace compounds we still haven't identified. Nature has been working on combining these in beneficial ways for all creatures for millions of years. Man has manufactured supplements—often isolated and sometimes synthetic—for less than 100 years. Do you really think that these can replace natural foods and natural supplements?

We know it seems preposterous, but, once again, regular bagels are not a health food because most are made of white flour. They are preferred over doughnuts or danish, but not over whole-wheat toast.

Energy bars and gels have a use for athletes. They are portable, convenient, nutritionally balanced and calorie-controlled. Raisins, dried apricots and peanuts aren't similarly measured. Both provide complex carbohydrates. In training and racing you want a quick conversion to usable energy with minimum energy expenditure for digestion. (Energy bars have a poor nutrition-to-dollar ratio. When a race supplies bars, gels, and nutritional drinks, that is immaterial.)

Eat or drink in small, frequent doses to keep your stomach filling and emptying: sip, rather than gulp; nibble rather than wolf down. That's an advantage of a "camel-back" water carrier, but, except on a bike, it is heavy.

Your digestive system is your body's fuel tank. The glycogen in your muscle can be loaded, but during a long event it needs reloading through your fuel tank. However, you can overload. Washing down a high-calorie gel (200 calories) with a high-calorie energy drink (another 200) can slow gastric emptying (how fast food leaves your stomach—where little absorption takes place—and enters your small intestine—where most absorption takes place).

Intake fat and protein, which take longer to digest than carbohydrate, on events of more than two hours. On shorter events, fat and protein are inefficient in refueling. As time stretches out, however, these give a more stable energy supply than simple carbohydrates.

Very simply, you can find the right combination in bars, gels, and commercial drinks or in foods from your kitchen. Experiment and mix it up. Some gels have no fat and no protein. They are great for quick energy; not so great for long events. Some gels have a goodly amount of both. So, of course, does a peanut butter and jelly sandwich. Raisins are as high in carbohydrates as candy bars with half the calories.

Balance your needs—quick, high-glycemic index foods

(chiefly the simple sugars) with foods with more complex carbohydrates and even with protein and fats for slow, steady gastric emptying. Remember that in most events, your body will use stored supplies—mostly fat.

For a competition longer than two hours, carbo loading more sophisticated than a pre-race spaghetti dinner is in order. Until recently, serious carbo loading was a long, hard routine. It began at least two weeks before a race and involved such a deprivation of carbohydrates that few accomplished it successfully.

More recently, sports research has settled on a far less arduous, week-long program that coincides with the pre-race training taper.

FOR THE IRONMAN OR IRONMAN DISTANCE

On prerace day six (the Sunday before the Saturday race) begin to drain stored muscle and liver glycogen. Liver stores go quickly; the muscle stores more slowly. Take your 60% carbohydrates to 10%. Replace 15% of this with protein, which means you'll cut caloric intake drastically. That's all right because you are tapering. If you are starving, take in a little fat with your protein so it stays in your stomach longer.

Also cut your training in half on pre-day six and go easy at that. Because this is low impact, it will begin to clear out carbohydrate stores.

On day five continue the same, but again cut your work-out. To your body this begins to look like starvation. It needs carbohydrates; it isn't getting them. It's getting protein instead. Protein isn't good for storage and recall. Protein, however, will keep your energy up during this depletion period.

This will not last, but if you again feel like you are starving —because while building endurance and speed, you were consuming enough calories to feed a passel of dwarfs—stuff yourself with celery, lettuce, summer squash, cucumbers, cabbage, radishes, and other zero foods (very low in calories, carbohydrates and protein—yet with fiber, vitamins and minerals).

On pre-day four, begin loading. By starving yourself of carbohydrate, you have made your body believe that famine came to the land. Now it has shifted into its anti-famine mode. Carbohydrates is what it needs to guard against starvation and it will take every gram that comes through the fuel line and try to put it into the storage tanks (muscles and liver). Since you are tapering, you are cutting the amount of carbohydrate you burn, so your body will concentrate on storage.

'Tis better to feed a steady stream of carbohydrate nutrients, so graze your way through the next three days. If you load too much at one time, the body flushes the excess out of the system. Snack on high carb bars, natural sugars as in fruits, dried fruits and some vegetables (carrots, particularly). Breakfast on bran muffins (watch the fat content), whole grain cereals, and breads; lunch on pasta with a red sauce or a little olive-oil, garlic, and basil; dine on rice or pasta with a lean meat sauce or chicken or a grilled chicken Caesar salad and whole grain or corn bread. Do something Oriental with little meat and many stir fried vegetables over brown rice. Use sugared fruit in red wine for dessert.

All of this is easy these days in Kailua/Kona. Twenty years ago, it wasn't. Most of today's triathletes are housed in condominiums, rather than hotels. Our friend who began St. Louis athletes' participation in Hawaii recalls that from their hotel room, eating right wasn't simple. He steered his athlete friends to Izimi's, a Japanese restaurant on the hill of the Queen K highway enroute to Captain Cook (a village). Izimi's staff was used to Ironman visitors ordering four bowls of rice with every entree.

The Japanese restaurant was also a good place to avoid

the fats. Today, don't do candy bars, seafood cream sauces, whole milk, Ben and Jerry's, chocolate, guacamole. If you have 6% fat stores, you have enough stored fat to do an Ironman. You don't need to add any more to carry around for hours.

In Kailua/Kona today, the produce farmer's market (which used to be an ad hoc thing that occurred on Alii drive just past Kahalu'u Bay beach park—the best beginners' snorkeling beach on the face of the earth) operates two days a week downtown. It offers better buys for fruit and vegetable eaters than any of the three supermarkets. The supermarkets, however, also sell local produce. Remember, in Hawaii, everything—including pineapple—is more expensive than in the 48 contiguous states. Why this is also true of local produce is a mystery.

On day four also start some salt loading. You won't need gobs, but in this hot-weather race, you'll lose lots.

Trim your training another 20 minutes and do the same on day three. Push—do intervals—but keep it light. You have all you are going to get in endurance (aerobic fitness), but you can push speed to remind your body of what you are going to ask of it on race day. Just don't wring out the carbohydrate stores you're loading.

On pre-day three, keep up carbo loading. How you accomplish your training will depend on your age. If you are over 50, take this day off as well as countdown days two and one. If you are over 40, keep intense training to 30 minutes. You just want your body to know that you are going to continue your demands on it. If you are younger, do a little more, push a little harder but don't give in to the urge to try to improve on what you already have.

In all of this, alternate modes. Don't run hard after day four. Jog a little in the heat of the day, bike too. Save the swimming for closer to race day. The purpose of your workouts in these days is to keep your muscles loose—so stretching and yoga are surely in order. Get acclimated, check out your equipment and blow away the butterflies.

By the way, if one of these prerace days is travel, plan ahead to do sufficient carbo loading without loading fat. If you are skipping meals, graze. Airline food—sans first-class—isn't notorious for its richness or sufficiency, but it's generally balanced. To load on carbo, supplement it. Pack fruit, dried fruit, energy and cereal bars and sports drinks.

A word of caution in carbo loading. Stay away from high-glycemic foods. They do not lend themselves to storage as well as more complex, more fibrous, slower to digest carbohydrates. Save the baked potatoes for a steak dinner in celebration and the pizza for an after-the-race treat.

On countdown day two, give your body a real rest. Work out only to accomplish the above-mentioned objectives. Eat high carb, but watch the calories. Hold the beer; it has too many calories with those carbohydrates. Put away the tuna and canned salmon; you don't need their protein-sans-calories. You don't even need their good fats for a couple of days. Avoid heavy fat content.

On countdown day one, exercise to loosen up and ease tension. Stick with high carbohydrate foods your body can digest easily. This may mean high-glycemic index foods, so it's a good day to eat bananas, papaya and pineapple. Although avocados grow locally on beautiful waxy-leafed trees, on this day don't eat them; they have too much fat and that slows digestion.

For the Hawiian Ironman, Thursday is the carbo-load dinner of pastas and salads. It almost always includes pirogees (the maker is a consistent sponsor) and although these are a high-glycemic-index food, they are excellent for carbo loading.

On Saturday, the race starts at 7 a.m., but don't eat to carbo load within 15 hours of that. Remember an average meal will take nearly that long to get through your digestive system and turn into glycogen. Drink lots of fluid, take in salt and avoid foods such as beans and broccoli because they produce gas.

This isn't the time go out for strange food. Don't try Indian, Portuguese, Ceylonese, although these island restaurants are wonderful. Don't do a luau. This isn't even the time to try Hawaii's or Australia's or Japan's fresh seafood. It isn't the time for Billy Bob's barbecue up at Captain Cook above Kailua/Kona.

Go to bed early; save the alcohol. When you get up on race day, eat breakfast. Take in additional carbohydrates two hours before the race. No matter how you have tried to load, you haven't succeeded with the liver. Its glycogen is gone overnight. Have whole-wheat toast, light butter, jelly, fruit (bananas or papaya), a whole-grain cereal with skimmed milk, a cup of coffee (with caffeine). Hold it to a cup or two because although caffeine will slow glycogen depletion, it can interfere with hydration.

Top breakfast off with an energy bar if you can't otherwise get to about 800 calories. If you just can't calm your stomach and your nerves enough to eat real food, have a high-energy supplement laid out. Since the Kailua pier has long lines before it opens, the anxiety is likely to bring you there several hours before the gun. Take food along. You must have this carbohydrate.

If the race won't have a sports drink available at the start (many don't), tuck one into your gear and down it 15 minutes before the gun. You need another before you set out on the bike. Put it with your bike gear along with at least one energy bar. On the swim, you are putting in a half-hour to two hours that are nutrition-less.

ON THE BIKE AND RUN

Take in 200 to 300 calories an hour. Experiment in training. The bike leg is the best chance to load. You won't want much solid food on the run, but for a marathon at the end of that grueling day, you need nutrition. On the run, stick with gels and liquids.

On the bike if you can average 300 calories an hour do so. Take them in various forms (bars, gels, cookies, dried fruit, crackers, boiled new potatoes—Tim's favorite) and constantly. Put foods into your stomach in small amounts that empty quickly, eat or drink every 15 minutes. As Tim's favorite reveals, you want high-glycemic-index foods here. Anything with too much fiber, too little surface, too much fat will sit in your stomach.

By all means, experiment with as much variety as you can carry and tolerate; you will feel better. Carry some stuff with you on the bike to give you variety. In Hawaii, you can pick up *your* "special needs" bag at the bike turnaround at Havi (56 miles out over a black road in a black field and up a long gradual hill, often fighting crosswinds or headwinds). When you finally get off the bike, a volunteer will be standing in your path to the changing tent holding out *your* run bag. You packed these bags with gear and sustenance and turned them in the day before. On the Kailua/Kona pier, at Havi, and at the Kona Surf they appear magically.

Plan your nutrition ahead. Then use the bars, gel, drink, cookies, bananas, and bagels along the route for variety, but use them wisely. Don't overload; it can weigh you down or cause cramps.

If you are not completely exhausted as the race ends, you have messed up. Your goal was to load as much as you needed just to finish. Near the finish line, adrenalin will kick in and give you a little extra. If you have enough more kick than that, you should have pressed harder.

On the other hand, ending up with a wobbly neck and knees that feel like rubber is worse. Heaven forbid you do a Julie-Moss. It's ok to fall into the arms of a volunteer or a companion, but not to be carried off to the medical tent for rehydration. (Although in hot Hawaii, probably between 20 and 30% of the finishers will need IVs.) Many races are now weighing athletes before the event to compare that weight with the weight of finishers who show up at the medical site for rehydration. Rehydration aids recovery; every athlete recovers more quickly with it, so perhaps it's being overused. Race sponsors pay for that and are now discriminating to determine who *needs* it.

You can suffer excess hydration and, even on a hot day, become waterlogged. Don't. The excess fluid passing through your body carries away with it essential electrolytes and minerals. In rare cases, brain edema can occur leading to a coma or even death. However, it is far easier to underhydrate. By the time dehydration begins to shut down your system, it's too late. Practice; decide how much liquid you need. Then overdo it a little.

RECOVERY

Recent research says that after a race opens a two-hour window to speed recovery by glycogen synthesis. By four hours that window has closed. It opens almost immediately, surely by 30 minutes postrace.

We've long known that carbohydrate consumption begins muscle glycogen replacement, but only recently have researchers clearly identified the important part insulin and protein play in this.

A current school of diet nutrition has fixated on lowering insulin levels as a way to burn more fat. For athletes it says that 40% carbohydrate, 30% protein, 30% fat will slow glycogen depletion and thus extend endurance.

Maybe, probably not, but even if, it's a bad plan because it hinders recovery. Its science is shaky, at best. Insulin doesn't make people fat and reducing insulin doesn't make people thin, thinner, or fatigue resistant.

Insulin is an essential facilitator of glycogen replacement and muscle recovery. Released by the pancreas in response to carbohydrate digestion (raising the blood sugar level), insulin helps transport the carbohydrate (glucose) from the blood into the muscle cell. There it can be stored as glycogen.

Secondly, at the muscle site, insulin stimulates an enzyme called glycogen synthetase, which transforms glucose into glycogen (its usable storage form). So an athlete on a 40-30-30 diet to lower blood insulin levels, also has lowered his/her ability to replenish muscle glycogen stores.

On the other hand, in recovery, adding protein to carbohydrate (according to the American College of Sports Medicine testing the optimal ratio is one to four) stimulates insulin production and speeds recovery. There is apparently a rather thin line here in protein addition. Too much slows gastric emptying and thereby slows absorption (remember, nutrients are not absorbed in the stomach, but only in the small intestine). Four parts carbohydrate to one part protein seems to tread that line.

The science of this protein addition in recovery indicates that the protein actually can almost double insulin production. In addition a protein amino acid called arginine further speeds glycogen replacement.

Arginine's role is a little more obscure. After exercise, the arginine in protein allows the body to increase fat metabolism. As the body burns more fat for energy, it releases more carbohydrate for glycogen replacement. Arginine doesn't act directly on either insulin production or carbohydrate synthesis. It simply allows us to utilize more fat for energy and therefore to send more carbohydrates to the muscles.

Clearly, the manufacturers of sports drinks and bars have already synthesized recovery products—some in the correct ratio, some with too much protein. They are not all on top of this kind or research (although some are underwriters of the research).

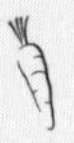

Key in recovery are two factors: when and what. The when is within two hours, the what is carbohydrate and protein intake on a four to one ratio.

As clearly, you can do this on your own with natural foods. Knowing exactly what your ratios are, however, will take some help and since ratio influences results, at present rely on the new recovery products—but check their ratios carefully; those we were given in 2000/2001 were too high in protein—or watch for information on how to do this naturally. Those formulations aren't as profitable, so they'll come slowly, but surely.

Chapter 12

Planning Training

If you are a Type A personality, competition will be the life-breath of your health program. You will have to know where you stand in physical fitness, as in every other aspect of your life. And you will work to excel.

A caution: Do not let this take over your life. Remember that you are doing this for longevity, quality of life and economic gain. What profit if you win medals but lose your soul?

You have a companion, children, parents, friends, work. Your health is important to every one of those people and to you, but it is not more important than they are. Everyone must understand always that your good health benefits them and, to some extent, will determine their success, as well as yours. That may not always be easy.

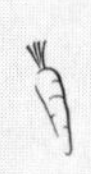

Post a sign on the refrigerator (or somewhere else obvious) that says, "My (mom, dad, husband, wife)'s good health benefits me, too. I will have him/her with me longer, and in the long run, it will make me healthier, wealthier and wiser."

We have a friend who began competing in triathlons locally and then nationally. He was married and had three still-small children. His job required long hours. It brought them a comfortable living with some surplus. When he began to train seriously, his wife felt that he was not holding up his share of child-rearing. He adjusted his training hours, giving up organized things that added hours to his day, but he also encouraged his wife and children to take up competition. They could train together.

The children did, won Ironkids age-group competition and the family traveled for their meets, as well as for his. Those accommodations worked well for years. Eventually, the children outgrew Ironkids and became high school athletes. By then, his wife, feeling that she had sacrificed some of her goals, went to work on education and a career.

It didn't work perfectly, but it worked. They spread the money and time they had to reach goals that took everyone's needs into consideration.

Set a goal, decide how much time, effort and money you can afford or are willing to devote to it and stick with it. For you, as for Ed Wolfgram and Tim Meyer, it might be easier to struggle than to succeed greatly. Success for many people is bait.

In 2000, following two years of trophying in his age group in Hawaii, Ed decided he had one more possibility of doing that before it became an age-factor long shot. He was 67. There were five Ironman qualifying spots in U.S. races for men 65 to 69. He came in second in his first race; the winner took the Ironman berth. Three weeks later in Lubbock, Texas, for the Buffalo Springs Lake half-Ironman competition, Ed was injured.

Fifteen miles into the 56-mile bike, as Ed came down a hill going 35 miles an hour, a triathlete coming out on the other side of the road swerved into Ed's lane. A head-on collision was coming. Ed hit the breaks to avoid that, flew over the handlebars heels over head. He landed on the right front of his helmet, shattering it, and skidded on his right shoulder to a stop on the road. On impact, the helmet crashed down on the bridge of his nose, bloodying it.

A good Samaritan stopped. He made sure Ed was conscious, had no broken bones, and wanted to continue. He made sure that the errant cyclist was off his bike without injury and coming up the ravine on Ed's side of the road. The Samaritan rode on.

After some time lapse that Ed wasn't fully aware of, he straightened up his handlebars and rode for 40 miles. Officials kept stopping him to be sure he could continue. By the time he finished the bike, he was an hour and a half behind his expected 5-hour-40-minute finish. He had little possibility of catching up, injured and bloodied as he was. He went to the medical tent instead of out on the run.

He lost his Ironman spot to a friend who finished in 6 hours and 30 minutes. Ed was too badly strained, scraped and bruised to do a full Ironman qualifying race six weeks later. That was to be his last shot at Hawaii that season. He asked the Ironman owners to give him a spot based on his record. They declined.

In response, he said to his wife, Dorothea, "Well, honey, I've had my years of priority. It's your turn. We'll go where you want, do what you want to do for the next two years. Then we're back on the circuit to race when I'm 70."

He set up other competitive goals. He won a spot on the U.S. Triathlon team for international competition in Edmonton, Alberta, in July 2001 and made that a long-term goal. He did well there. He did local competition and a marathon or two, but none dominate the Wolfgrams' life as Ironman competition does. After seven Ironman races in Hawaii in October, they are seeing other parts of the world for a while.

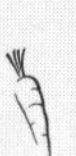

Keep your competition and goals in perspective. Balance them with the rest of your life. Occasionally, take a break to pay more attention to other things. Be aware of how your goal impacts other people and things that matter to you. However, keep those people aware of how your good health and competitive spirit benefit them too, now and for years to come.

PERIODIZATION

When you have set a goal and decided on the resources you need to and can give to it, set up a long-term training program. The best approach is to periodize your routine: set up a plan that changes your workouts at regular intervals to achieve goals of that period and work toward a long-term goal. It will probably be a year-long plan or longer.

It will help you cope with the physical and mental demands of intense training. Along the way, you will also be more satisfied because your workouts will not be the same forever. You will use variables such as the number of repetitions or the amount of weight, the exercises, the time spent or the rest periods needed. You could, of course, meet your long-term goal by perfectly balancing each workout, but that would lead to disaster. Imagine how boring it would be to do a perfect workout day in and day out without end. Don't.

Finally, periodization helps prevent injuries by not straining the same muscles endlessly day after day, week after week, month after month. Athletes who compete are often exercise-obsessed. They train through pain or, if they feel good, push harder and harder. Eventually, unless they plan change in advance, it comes in an unwelcome way: they are injured.

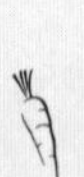

Injuries occur more frequently when you need rest, not more work. Periodization changes intensity and activity. If you have hit a training plateau, chances are that you need a change. Plateaus come when you have pushed and pushed and achieved and achieved, but in doing so you are in need of rest and recovery.

If you allow your body to do nothing in rest, it will lose some of what you have worked for. But if you switch to another training plane and retouch your base occasionally, it will recover and hold the gain.

The final beauty of periodization is that you tailor a program to fit your needs.

Now, you can do this alone, but it will be much easier, more effective and faster, to consult a professional. That will take preparation. Talk to your fellow athletes. Pick their brains. See what works for them and try it out a little bit.

Consult the literature. There are good articles on training programs every month in sports, training and fitness magazines and on Web sites. Since periodization is currently the rage under that name, all of them will use it.

If you consult a professional (a sports physiologist, a trainer, a successful coach—amateur or professional) sit down with him/her to make your goals and options clear. Decide what level of basic fitness you want to maintain. Explain your competitive goals and timing.

Periodization was discovered and used in the 1950s by exercise scientists and coaches from the former Eastern Bloc countries of the Soviet Union and East Germany. Until the West discovered its value, those athletes beat the socks off the world in many areas. Illegal drugs also played a part in the Soviet Bloc athletic success, but their training methods were far superior for some time.

Plan changes. Plan work. Plan rest. Then stick to that plan.

A periodized program has two variables: "training volume" —the total amount of training (miles ridden, run, swum, walked, skied, bladed, rowed, stepped, danced, weight lifted and so on); and "training intensity"—the difficulty of the segment. This can be time spent at a percentage of your heart max or some other intensity measure. For weight lifters, it is the number of repetitions as a percentage of the one-repetition maximum.

The standard American terminology for periods is "off season," "preseason," and "in-season." Each is self-explanatory, but "off" isn't off, it's reduced. It allows for rest and recovery and for other important parts of your life to come to the fore.

Use off-season for active recovery. Use other activities to maintain your base-level fitness. If you swim competitively and for that swim every day, drop back to three times a week, but vary your strokes now. In doing so, you build opposing muscles to stabilize the muscles you overuse in season. Take more hours at resistance training, do some running or walking, some golfing even. Active recovery keeps you energized and aerobically fit.

Professional athletes no longer come to training camp overweight and out of shape. Coaches won't put up with it. They want the preseason time they pay for to be used to bring their athletes to a high level of training and cooperation fast. Amateur coaches don't like it either and often simply cut an out-of-shape contender from the roster early. You have a coach too. Don't put up with it in yourself.

The length of each period depends on the length of the competitive season, but it also depends on your base fitness level and your age. At 16, getting ready for a sport may take a few weeks. At 50, bringing your body up to peak isn't that easy. For an adult athlete, preseason lasts two to four months; sometimes more. Don't push; that can lead to injury.

Preseason begins sport-specific training in earnest again. In the beginning plan high volume, low intensity. Concentrate on skill work. For swimming, re-perfect your stroke and your kick for competition, but don't abandon other strokes or pulls. In tennis spend more hours on the court, but don't abandon the resistance workouts to keep opposing knee and elbow muscles strong.

As the competitive season approaches, the volume of training will decrease and intensity increase. Also, the volume of skill training will increase.

The goal of preseason is to bring you into competition at peak. Remember, the first races, matches, meets count as much as the last. In addition, being ready gives you the great advantage of being ready; other competitors aren't always. If your program is well planned and executed, you'll have the same advantage at the season's end. Some competitors who haven't planned and executed well will suffer fatigue.

Periodization takes a long, careful, calculated look at what you need to meet a seasonal goal. It sets up activities, volume, and intensity. The best periodization is pretty rigid. Remember, it's not calculated to how you are doing or feeling on or in any particular day, week, month, but on a slow steady progression—which will always have some plateaus.

In-season can be straightforward or complicated. For the Ironman competition in Hawaii, for instance, it's not simple. Any competition that requires qualifying requires complex periodization.

The Hawaiian competitors who get there by winning a qualifying spot peak for qualifying races and then plan leeway to rest, relax, and recuperate and really peak for the October competition. In addition, periodization for the Ironman is complicated by the length and condition of the qualifying race: events will be half or full distance; cool, moderate or hot; flat or hilly. Those conditions change the goals and therefore the periodization, but the October race is always the ultimate goal.

Any competition that depends on racking up points or scores for an ultimate competition complicates periodization. So does competition that successively qualifies winners for a local, state, regional, national, international competition.

Yet periodization not only works for all of them; it gives the competitor an edge because it's planned and executed with individual, specific goals in mind. Winning competitors don't make spur-of-the-moment decisions—those can result in injury. Plan a year; Olympic hopefuls periodize years.

For some purposes, European terminology may be helpful. It speaks of: "Preparation"—off-season; "first transition"—preseason; "competition"—in-season; "second transition" an aftermath off-season. The second transition is a let-down for physical and mental recovery. It usually is not sufficient to maintain a high level of basic fitness. That comes in "Preparation."

To construct a periodized program without professional aid, find and use examples in books, periodicals on the Internet. Then individualize.

Chapter 13

Wrapping It All Up

To get ready for the Ironman in Hawaii, Ed Wolfgram trains three hours a day, six days a week. In the U.S., qualifying events for the world championship in Hawaii usually begin in the spring. His serious training starts in January; the race is in October.

That leaves him two months to goof off a little. It is his "off-season." So he trains three hours a day, but he eats a little more, gains a few pounds, and degenerates a little. In a way it's again Freud's "regression in service to the ego." He falls off the wagon so that he can stay on most of the time by looking forward to falling off again.

We are not necessarily advocating that regime. Off-season can be a time when training takes less time and other parts of your life can consume more.

For athletes with children, that may be the time that saves your marriage. Sometimes, however, more leisure time can be like Viagra (figuratively, perhaps not literally). If your spouse has a routine that runs smoothly without you when you are training hard, finding you more available could be discombobulating.

Ed keeps the three-hour routine because then he doesn't have to struggle to reclaim those hours. Obeying somebody's law, his tasks expand to fill the time available. When an hour for exercise slips away, it's hard to wrestle it back. In addition, since the majority of his exercise time is early—5:30-8:30 a.m.—keeping the same pace jibes with his sleep patterns.

By his routine, Ed has persevered and satisfied his competitive spirit. Despite some minor bike accidents, he has been essentially injury free for 20 years. There are lessons to be learned from his routine. Those have been said more than once in this book, but let's reiterate.

Lessons 1 *Be social.* Make a major part of your program of physical activity a social event, as well as a health event.

Lesson 2 *Cross-train.* Otherwise, you are courting disabling injury. Make up a program that suits your lifestyle and preferences but uses various major muscle groups.

Lesson 3 *Practice yoga.* There may be other ways to achieve balance and flexibility, but yoga is the time-tested, time-honored, body-balanced practice that stretches and relaxes. For those who practice seriously, it is magic.

Lesson 4 *Do resistance training* with Nautilus or free weights. Aerobic exercise for the heart was the message of the '60s, '70s, and '80s. Resistance training was the message of the '90s. Even in experiments with the frail and the elderly, training with Nautilus and free weights never failed to strengthen the muscles stressed.

The sum of the above builds muscle and overall body strength, endurance and flexibility. These are the bottom line of fitness. Barring serious illness or accident, there is nothing else between you and 100 years except good nutrition, abstinence of tobacco and other drugs and spare use of alcohol. (We are assuming that you have good genes. Most of us do and those who don't improve their chances of leading a long, healthful, active life with these practices.)

You do not have to belong to a health club, YMCA, community recreation center, or other established facilities to maintain fitness, but it surely helps. These offer organized programs, as well as facilities and equipment. Unless you are so isolated you cannot use a fitness center regularly, don't fail to do so.

In the U.S., these are the boon of the past several decades, although the trend began 100 years earlier. Now it's hard to find a neighborhood, a suburb, a small town without a recplex. And it is hard to travel long in an urban area without finding a small private, for-profit fitness center.

We have a young Ironwoman friend who lives on a small Caribbean island. She designs her own training program with an at-home gym because finding programs and facilities is difficult. Yet she has found training partners because they are a necessity. When she comes back to St. Louis, she immediately plugs into the training network. These exist in every community, find them!

If you cannot, make them up, even if your groups starts as a twosome. No matter what your level, health-conscious partners are absolutely essential for motivation, companionship and competition.

If some parts of your routine are solo, think about getting a dog. There is no more eager, appreciative and accommodating partner. John Muir, the great naturalist and conservationist, explored glaciers in Alaska. A lonely task, one would think, but his 1879 voyage, during which he found and mapped Glacier Bay, was shared with a dog. He wrote once of its heroics, relating that from the time they left camp until they returned, he kept up a steady dialogue with his four-legged friend and his friend responded.

Faithfulness, however, is a dog's absolute. More than once, if Muir's day was to be on sharp ice, he tried to sneak out of camp without the pup. He never succeeded. They once returned with the dog's bloody paws wrapped in Muir's shredded shirt. When a friend of ours cannot take his dog running, he must sneak out. He keeps several small bags in which he hides his running shoes because they are his dog's signal. Our friend's family complains that without the deceit, the dog mourns for hours.

It is so much easier to be faithful to your exercise, if someone else is counting on you. It is so much harder to roll over and go back to sleep. Besides, these are often people who share other life goals with you. Some become good friends.

If you compete, you will find a built-in network. You train together. You root for friends, they root for you. Even if you haven't shared a particular event, you may spend hours finding out how it went.

Competition is like life. There are people you dislike and love to beat (and that is motivating) and people who are always gracious. For good sports, every level of competition builds friendships. Going to an event is like going to a reunion. The more you participate, the more your circle widens. It's wonderful. And so self-selective, it's often matchmaking. Be aware of how many professional athletes marry other athletes.

CROSS-TRAINING

Ed Wolfgram counts the day he discovered triathlons as the day that initiated his longevity as an endurance athlete. Prior to that he had been a runner for exercise and a biker for transport.

The latter began with our decision to live in the city close to our work. In 1965, Ed moved into a new city highrise and bought bicycles. For him, it was faster and less hassle to get to the university hospitals by bicycle than by auto. So compact was our neighborhood, in pre-bicycle days Ed sometimes "lost" his car. He would take it someplace in the neighborhood and, without thinking about how he came, walk from there to home, hospital or office. A few years later we bought a city home nearby.

As the months went by, Ed's bicycle range increased with his endurance. So did our German shepherd's. The dog—who was so massive obedience training was a necessity—ran dutifully next to Ed's left pedal. Ed's legs became stronger; the dog's chest filled out. A friend once said, "Nobody who hears that bark is going to come to investigate."

By the time Ed took up running, he was a 60-mile a week cyclist, but that wasn't keeping the weight off. He began running because it was the most efficient use of his exercise time. He had run for five years (including two Boston marathons) and cycled for 15 before he discovered the triathlon; but he was a head-above-the-water swimmer. He joined a sunrise fitness swim (6 a.m. three days a week).

As he practiced these sports, he discovered that the balance kept him more pain-free than he had been previously. The nagging pain in a football-injured knee abated somewhat. The soreness in the neck, experienced in trying to keep a bicycle tuck position, lessened because he was building neck muscle by swimming. The minor leg stress pain experienced after hard runs, stopped threatening to disable him. Not only was he running less, he was building muscles antagonistic to running muscles by learning to pull up on the bicycle pedals, as well as push down. Running was calf-intensive; cycling was thigh-intensive; swimming was upper-body-intensive. It made a nice complementary package.

It all began to work together coordinately because despite the fact that he was putting in more hours, he was using various muscle groups. Had he not increased his exercise hours, he would have achieved a far healthier routine through the variety alone. Eventually, he added Nautilus work to the end of his University-based swim program.

"The body is really no stronger than its weakest link, so I work primarily on those weak links—my neck, elbows, knees, shins. And I work out body balance. Since I'm right handed, I have a whole body right dominance. At the machines, I do more left side repetitions than right to compensate for that."

Cross-training doesn't mean swim, bike, run, although that is a proven way to balance various muscle groups. If you are not competing, make up your own regimen: walk, bike, do some upper-body weight work; walk, bike, play tennis and golf; bike, blade, play handball or racquet ball; play golf, baseball, bike; surf, play volleyball, jog; row (or kayak), do Nautilus, walk or run. Always, however, do some resistance work and stretch.

There is no magic in three except that two is probably too few to prevent injury through variety. And four or five may be too many to keep balanced on a regular basis. However, find a cross-train combination that suits you and design a balanced program around it.

Remember you are looking for physical activity that is cardiovascular, but that is not "exercise" exclusive. We have a friend who stays trim and healthy by refereeing and doing a little weight work. An 80-year-old friend loses pounds every spring when she can get into the garden. Her challenge was to find an indoor activity for the winter months, so she mall walks and does her own housework, but hires help when she'd rather spend her time gardening and swimming. Another busy physician never uses the elevator in her hospitals; she walks up and down. She says it takes absolutely the same amount of time. For upper-body work she swims and does Nautilus. Our neighbor teaches dance, swims and gardens ferociously. She runs some with Ed in the winter. Some elderly friends dance and walk. Ed talked them into some home exercise equipment.

Be careful in making up your cross-training program that you are not heavily into sports that are hard on your joints. Tennis is notoriously so because of its quick moves and pivots that strain both elbows and knees. Soccer is the same for ankles and knees. Basketball has the same pitfalls, and then adds the perils of falls onto a hard surface. Rugby speaks for itself so far as tough moves, falls, bangs. Football is great so long as it's flag and does not involve tackles.

But some of these sports may be important to you. They are fun, take skill and are competitive. Don't give them up. Just don't overdo. Balance them with activities that strengthen other muscle groups and, to be really safe, do some resistance work to strengthen at-risk parts.

YOGA

All exercisers need to stretch to maintain flexibility and balance. Yoga is a several-thousand year old program that organizes stretching and balancing to make it a body art. For those who practice regularly, it also brings relief from tension. The very quietness of the art promotes serenity. The variety of asnas (poses) covers every muscle, joint and organ from fingers and toes to hamstring and abdominal muscles.

In yoga you learn to listen to your own body. There are several forms of yoga practiced. Choose one that suits your circumstances and personality.

Once again, it's surely possible to practice yoga individually. Books, tapes, and videos abound. However, it's now pretty easy to make it a social event. You are also more likely to stick with it if you go with a partner. There is some group energy generated in a yoga practice that benefits all and most classes are held in spaces that minimize distraction and promote concentration. Frequently, membership in a yoga center is inexpensive, but health clubs and community centers often invite members to participate in yoga sessions free or at a small cost.

Judge a yoga instructor by how his/her program uses the tried and true postures such as bends, twists, lifts and inversions for a whole-body workout that avoids harmful stress. A good instructor also will have a bag of tricks to modify poses to begin where each student is and work from there. That is the beauty of a yoga practice; where you are (no matter how flexible or inflexible) is exactly where you should be.

Like many of the Asian practices, yoga is somehow more than the sum of its parts. Tai chi may be an acceptable substitute. So may aikido or karate. Ask around, try different routines if yoga is not your cup of tea. We have friends who find it much too laid back for tolerance.

There is a simple yoga routine called the Salute to the Sun (designed for morning but effective any time) that can be an effective 10-minute warm up or a slower, relaxing workout.

The salute can be done slowly and deliberately, holding poses for a few moments before going on to the next. That resembles tai chi in its fluidity; however, the downward dog pose is a power pose that requires strength so the routine is not as simple as it looks.

SALUTE TO THE SUN YOGA ROUTINE

Begin facing east to salute the sun. Stand relaxed with hands in front in a prayer position.

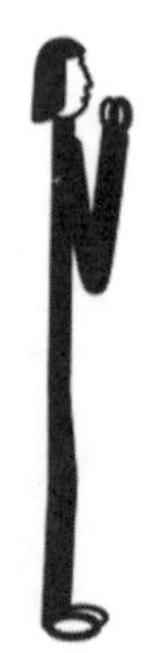

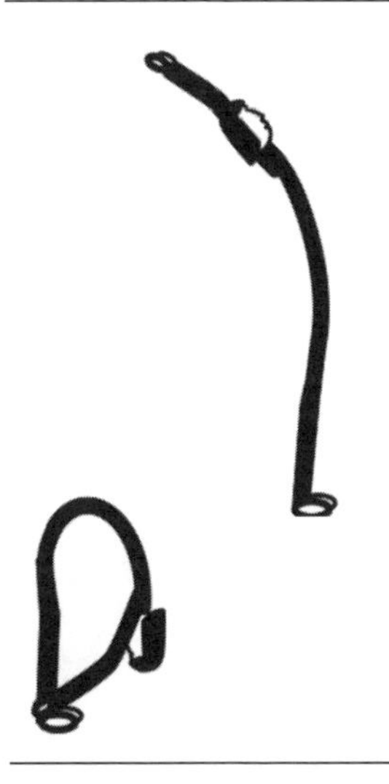

Reach up, spread arms, reach back, come forward to touch toes.

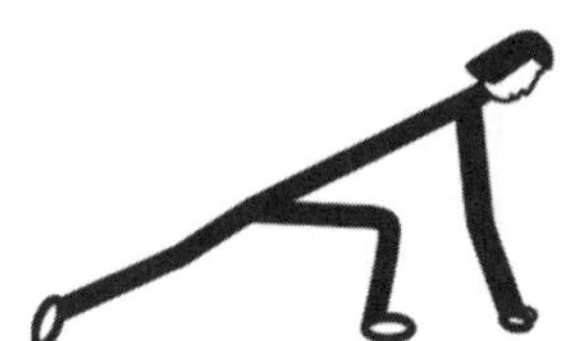

With hands flat on floor, stretch right leg back into a lunge position. Chin up, back straight.

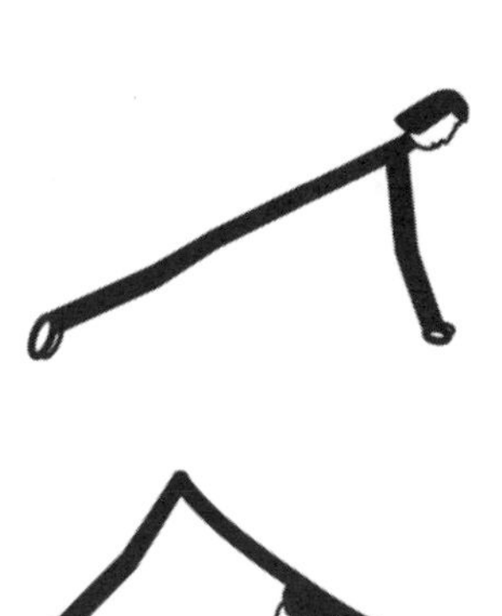

Left leg back, shift weight equally to feet and hands, feet and hands flat, arms straight (the isosceles triangle down-face dog, in yoga parlance).

Drop to knees. Then come up on toes. Swoop forward parallel to floor, forearm stiff. To end up forearm stiff, weight on toes and palms.

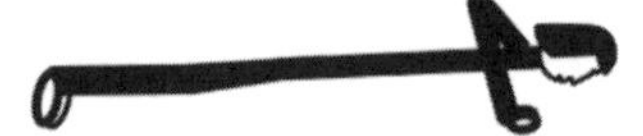

Come up on arms, tuck feet.

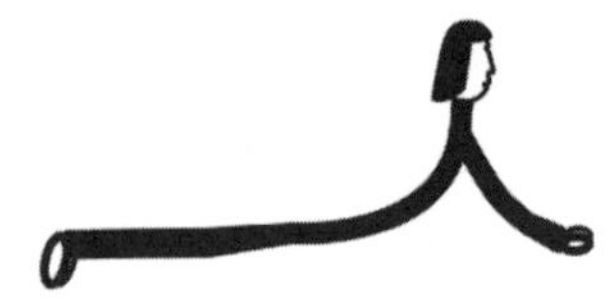

Lifting body with arms, shift weight back to downface dog, feet flat.

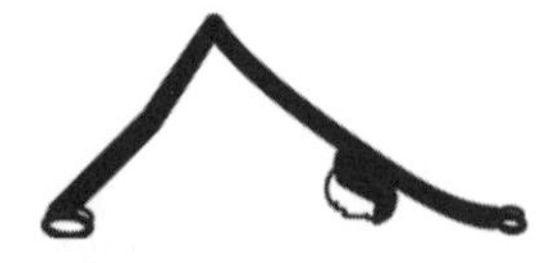

Pull right leg forward into lunge position.

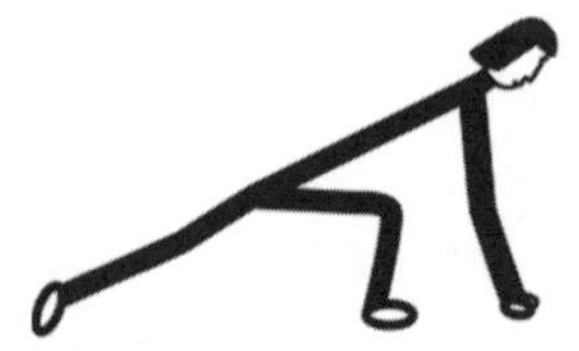

Advance left leg, hands flat on floor.

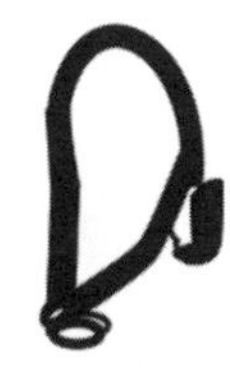

Stand up with arms out, bring them back apart, bring them to prayer position overhead.

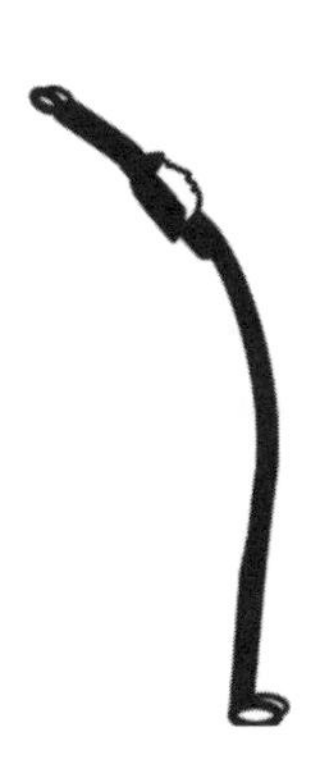

Return to standing pose. Pause.

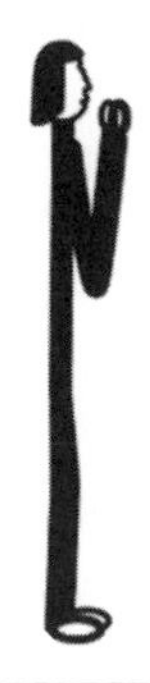

[Repeat leading with left leg.]

It can also, however, be done quickly, as a calisthenic. After two or three repetitions, it will leave you breathless, but awakened. Do at least three sets at a time.

Use the salute as it fits your need. On a frosty morning it will quickly warm you up and loosen you up. Later in the day, it can slowly calm and relax you.

Yoga will help avoid injury. Never, however, if you are injured, try to press away pain. Relent. Rest. Then come back gradually as you heal.

RESISTANCE TRAINING

Finally, either buy some home equipment, join a gym, or settle for a set of weights to do strength training. If you do it daily, your program can be a little as 15 minutes. Television is the perfect accompaniment. If you watch the news every night, make it a habit to do so at least several nights a week while you go through your routine. If you are a sports fan, pull up the rowing machine or the bicycle, oil them up to be silent, and do double duty. If you watch videos, hook up the VCR in the exercise space and vary your activity throughout.

Weights are surely the easiest equipment to handle and the most flexible and cheapest. A Nautilus machine is always a good investment if you use it. So is a bike, a rowing machine, a cross-country skier, a piece of ab equipment.
In all cases it might be a good idea to consult an exercise physiologist, a trainer, a physical therapist to have a program designed specifically for you. Remember, you want maximum flexibility to avoid being bored and maybe giving up.

If resistance training weren't so easy to combine with the sedentary activities of your life, we'd say make it a social event. That works best for some people. Do what works for you, but do it.

Our son Kurt is, for all, an encouraging example of his father's wisdom and philosophy. From age 8, Kurt was an

AAU (Amateur Athletic Union) swimmer. He swam throughout his high school years. He carried his exercise habits with him to college, but his small school did not have a swim team. Still he ran and did some Nautilus work.

When he began law school, his physical fitness fell apart. He simply didn't have time for it. Yet, he managed to swim 45-minutes twice a week. "It wasn't enough to keep the weight off or my body in good condition, but it relieved the stress and quieted me mentally and emotionally."

After law school, back in St. Louis and working at a law firm, he joined his father at morning swim and he and his wife bicycled on weekends. His weight came down and his muscles tightened. He competed occasionally in triathlons. Then came one child, a house, two more children, and the task of building his solo law practice. Disaster!

Yet at 33, he realized that fitness was essential to every aspect of his life. For his wife, children, profession, he says, he needs to feel as good as he did when he was that high school athlete.

He has restructured his day to plug into or arrange early-morning biking with friends. He is running some, but going easy on an Achilles tendon weakness. He is swimming regularly at a new YMCA near his house. And he is watching his weight. Years ago, he forsook the chewing tobacco that was his high-school-crowd's machismo.

He says, "I've discovered that those who influence our lifestyle the most are our peers. Strange as it may seem, choosing friends, companions, models wisely will be among the most important *health* decisions we will ever make."

Fitness does not start with exercise. It starts with the decision that its place in your life is central.

The PBS show *Nova* takes us regularly and routinely to worlds beyond our world. We know that we occupy a unique and essential place in the whole order. Mapping the human genome has taught us the connectedness of our inner world. We do not stand apart from universal order. We are in it and it is in us.

"As a psychiatrist," Ed says, °"I try to teach people to view their own mortality in that light. What we do, what we teach, who we are is essentially a part of the tide of human experience. How we conduct our lives sends ripples out to infinity. None of us can measure our influence. It is boundless. In that sense, we are immortal."

Disclaimer

Before undertaking any strenuous exercise program or sport, always consult your doctor. Between you, assess the appropriateness in light of your medical condition, history, and medication regimen. If you are receiving medical treatment for any chronic illness, consult your doctor about *any* new exercise stress. Always go slowly and be cautious.

Nutritional and therapeutic opinions stated here are based on our experience and reading. Research is ongoing.

Over and over again as
Ed Wolfgram spoke on
fitness to St. Louis area
groups, listeners said,
"You should write a book."

So we did.

To contact Ed

email: dorawolfgram32@aol.com

website: www.fitness-never2late.com

address: Ed Wolfgram
14 Hortense Place
St. Louis, Missouri 63108

phone: 314-367-1944 (*office*)